D1193666

Praise for *Food Ji*

This book will help many people with every
all start with the same premise. We who eat too much, too often, and who
find ourselves fat, miserable, bulimic, unhealthy, or just wanting to lose 20
pounds before Christmas are in the same boat. Dr. Tarman's book shows
how many ways there are to get help and get healed. My own solution —
through the twelve steps of GSA — presents the approach that has saved
my life — that we — all of us, just alcoholics — are allergic to sugar, grains,
flour, wheat, and corn! — yes, all grains! — the same ingredients that are
in alcohol. Avoiding these foods and eating three weighed meals a day
and nothing in between can lead you to find the last house on the block,
which is a mansion!

— Judy Collins, singer, songwriter, and author
of *Cravings: How I Conquered Food*

Dr. Vera Tarman aptly takes the science of sugar addiction and draws a
convincing clinical profile of the sugar/food addiction syndrome. With
plenty of clinical scenarios, Dr. Tarman illustrates and explains the various
stages of food addiction. She then shows how food addiction recovery is
possible and sustainable in the long term. *Food Junkies* is a must read for
patients, students, and clinicians interested in addiction medicine and/
or obesity management.

— Dr. Nicole Avena, research scientist and assistant professor at
Princeton University and Mount Sinai School of Medicine and
author of *Why Diets Fail (Because We Are Addicted to Sugar)*

For all those who have struggled with weight loss and failed, here is a
wise book that applies the addiction model to food. Tarman tackles the
neurobiology of pleasure and the epidemic of obesity and makes sense of
both. With a no-nonsense approach, Tarman offers a thoughtful, ground
breaking exploration of a subject that plagues the majority of readers.

— Ann Dowsett Johnston, author of *Drink: The Intimate
Relationship Between Women and Alcohol*

As someone who regularly treats patients suffering from food addiction and someone who has recovered from it, Dr. Tarman is the quintessential expert on food addiction. This book is a must read for anyone struggling with a food addiction.

— Chef A.J., author of *The Secrets to Ultimate Weight Loss*

Dr. Vera Tarman brings together in this book knowledge of physiology and the brain, experience of treatment for addiction, and sensitivity to the nature of food addiction. She takes us through the process of understanding, enlightenment, and finally hope.

— Esther Helga Guðmundsdóttir, director of INFACT International School for Food Addiction Counselling and Treatment

Are you one of those people who thinks food addiction isn't real? Then you might be what Dr. Vera Tarman describes in her book as a food junkie! I was addicted to sugar and other processed carbohydrates over a decade ago and found my way back to health and recovery thanks to some basic lifestyle changes that made me whole again. Dr. Tarman walks you through all the necessary steps to make that happen for you, too. Addiction is real, but it's not inevitable. Grab back control of your health now!

— Jimmy Moore, author of *Cholesterol Clarity and Keto Clarity*

FOOD
JUNKIES

RECOVERY FROM FOOD ADDICTION

FOOD JUNKIES

VERA TARMAN, MD | SECOND EDITION

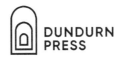

DUNDURN
PRESS

Copyright © Vera Tarman, 2019

All rights reserved. No part of this publication may be reproduced, stored in a retrieval system, or transmitted in any form or by any means, electronic, mechanical, photocopying, recording, or otherwise (except for brief passages for purpose of review) without the prior permission of Dundurn Press. Permission to photocopy should be requested from Access Copyright.

Cover designer: Laura Boyle | Cover image: © Ocean Photography

Library and Archives Canada Cataloguing in Publication

Tarman, Vera Ingrid, author
Food junkies : recovery from food addiction / Vera Tarman, MD. --
Second edition.

Includes bibliographical references and index.
Issued in print and electronic formats.
ISBN 978-1-4597-4197-3 (softcover).--ISBN 978-1-4597-4198-0 (PDF).--
ISBN 978-1-4597-4199-7 (EPUB)

1. Eating disorders. 2. Compulsive eating. I. Title.

RC552.E18T37 2019 616.85'26 C2018-905372-0
C2018-905373-9

Conseil des Arts du Canada Canada Council for the Arts Canada ONTARIO ARTS COUNCIL CONSEIL DES ARTS DE L'ONTARIO an Ontario government agency un organisme du gouvernement de l'Ontario

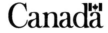

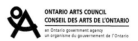

We acknowledge the support of the Canada Council for the Arts, which last year invested $153 million to bring the arts to Canadians throughout the country, and the Ontario Arts Council for our publishing program. We also acknowledge the financial support of the Government of Ontario, through the Ontario Book Publishing Tax Credit and Ontario Creates, and the Government of Canada.

Nous remercions le Conseil des arts du Canada de son soutien. L'an dernier, le Conseil a investi 153 millions de dollars pour mettre de l'art dans la vie des Canadiennes et des Canadiens de tout le pays.

Care has been taken to trace the ownership of copyright material used in this book. The author and the publisher welcome any information enabling them to rectify any references or credits in subsequent editions.
— *J. Kirk Howard, President*

The publisher is not responsible for websites or their content unless they are owned by the publisher.

Dundurn Press
Toronto, Ontario, Canada
dundurn.com, @dundurnpress

TO CATHY SCHWARTZ,
MY BELOVED PARTNER.
MAY WE LIVE HAPPILY EVER AFTER.

CONTENTS

PREFACE TO THE SECOND EDITION

Since I wrote the first edition of *Food Junkies* in 2014, much has changed — and little has changed. This new edition includes the most promising current research and details the latest advances in clinical practices and treatments, including my own. We may still have a long way to go, but giant steps have been taken in some areas. And many of the people I interviewed earlier have successfully navigated the minefields of food sobriety. I also bring their stories up to date.

First, the hopeful news: In the last four years, our awareness of how specific foods (such as sugar) ensnare both the hormonal appetite regulators and the reward circuitry of the brain has grown exponentially. Studies highlighting how sugar can be addictive are cited continually in the media.

Growing numbers of consumer groups are aghast at how the food industry is manipulating our appetites for its own profit. Calls to regulate the food industry and legislate healthy eating are multiplying. There are Internet chat groups, summits, cookbooks, and public lectures offering to help people quit sugar and other addictive foods. The tipping point of awareness that we need to stem the tide of addictive foods is approaching.

While we agree that some foods, such as sugar, are addictive, the bad news is that we are loath to recognize the dynamic of addiction that other foods ignite. Even clinicians scoff at this biological imperative, unwilling to identify the withdrawal and lack of choice that eating some foods engender. This unwillingness means that diagnosis, research, and funding of treatment of food addiction continues to flounder. When it comes to acknowledging the syndrome of food addiction, we remain in the dark ages.

I am unable to be objective about food addiction. I have struggled with this disease for decades, so, although my purpose in this book is to present a fact-based examination of food addiction, I can hardly be neutral.

Many of us have struggled to control our addiction through diet pills, diet doctors, and even diet candy.[1] We have spent thousands of dollars on Weight Watchers and Jenny Craig, therapists and psychiatrists, weight-loss vitamins and herbs. We have ingested diuretics, laxatives, and other substances to purge ourselves of extra food. We have exercised hours each day, so obsessively that we eliminated the rest and relaxation most people enjoy on weekends and vacations.

Our eating has been out of control; we've often ingested enough calories in an hour to fuel a two-hundred-pound male for days. We have repeatedly tried, and failed, to tame our appetites. We have enlisted people — friends, family, even professionals — to help us by shaming, blaming, bribing, nagging, cajoling, ignoring, encouraging, comforting, and punishing.

A food addict myself, I am on a passionate mission to present vital information to the many individuals who struggle with unwanted eating behaviours. I want to give readers a better understanding of the continuum that begins with food compulsions and ends with full-blown addiction.

For years, food addicts of all types — including myself — tried to talk about this phenomenon, but all too often our disclosures were met with light-hearted dismissals (*Oh, everyone eats a little too much sometimes*) or blunt skepticism (*It's not a disease, you know; you just eat too much*). Now that obesity, one of the hallmark symptoms of food addiction, has grown to epidemic proportions, scientists and medical professionals are no longer laughing. Instead, they are taking a closer look at what is really going on in the bodies and brains of those of us who struggle with our food intake. In *Food Junkies*, I present this information about the addictive nature of food in a format that can be understood by patients, clinicians, and, most importantly, the general public. And I introduce you to people who are struggling with this disease and tell their stories — their tragedies and victories — which have been for so long silenced, scoffed, scorned.

I don't want the book to be drily academic, the sort written by experts dispensing prescriptive advice. Though you will find helpful information here, much of it drawn from authoritative studies, the book also contains very personal stories — moving accounts full of feeling and struggle. Given my history as both a food addict and a clinician in the addiction field, I am well situated to present this information in an authentic, accessible way. As yet, there have been no books like mine, written by an author who has both experienced food addiction and its recovery and who is also equipped to speak from the authoritative stance of a medical clinician in the field.

In this book you will meet men and women suffering from food compulsions and addictions as well as those who have recovered. You will also meet people who are not addicted to food, but who have a tendency to overeat. Although their names have been changed, they are all real people whom I have met in my practice. You will meet Mary, who made the decision to lose weight when her scale indicated that she weighed more than two hundred pounds. She has managed to keep her weight off for many years. And you'll meet Janet, who insists that her lack of willpower is her real problem; she has lost weight and kept it off, but she is only able to do so as long as she sticks to her diet. And you'll also meet Ellen, who, despite great willpower, simply cannot control her bingeing at night. She worries that she might be a food addict.

You will be introduced to Laura, who is addicted to alcohol as well as food. While she no longer drinks, she simply cannot stop eating. As badly as she wants to stop, her cravings for food are even stronger than her cravings for alcohol. You'll learn about Lawrence, a morbidly obese food addict, whose death marks the inevitable conclusion of this disease when left untreated. And you'll meet Ruthann, whose primary addiction is *undereating*. Yes, I believe that even anorexics suffer from a kind of food addiction. Ruthann learns to control her anorexia by applying the same approaches I present for food addicts who overeat to her undereating patterns.

I have interviewed clinicians who have stepped outside the box, experimenting with treatment approaches for eating disorders. Among them is Renae Norton, who has treated hundreds of anorexics and bulimics and has concluded that both groups achieved recovery only when they abstained from all drugs, alcohol, *and* specific trigger foods. (If they didn't, she found, her clients would eventually relapse, with each relapse harder to recover from.) Connie Stapleton is another psychologist who works specifically with post-bariatric patients to ensure that the weight they lose through surgery is not regained by eating addictively in the months following the surgery.

Finally, you will meet people who have found effective solutions for themselves. Martha, for example, has stopped eating sugar and flour, and now weighs and measures her food down to the last ounce. Despite inquiring looks from others, she brings a scale to every restaurant meal. Once one hundred pounds overweight, she has kept the extra weight off for more than twenty years. More important, Martha has finally found a level of contentment with her eating. She provides a message of hope that freedom from food cravings is possible. For Martha, this freedom is so delicious that it overrides any pleasure that the food might have given.

My message is simple: If you see yourself as a food addict, you must treat your trigger foods as a drug. The most successful treatment for any drug addiction, from alcohol to drugs to food, is abstinence from the trigger substance. Our addicted brain — whether it is for genetic, psychological, or even environmental reasons — *is wired to crave more as soon as even the smallest amount has entered our system.* Like a flame igniting kindling, trigger foods ignite a fiery and voracious appetite that makes us want to eat, eat, eat.

While the message in this book may be simple, it's not an easy one. The message of abstinence from a drug of choice is a hard one to hear, especially since so many otherwise excellent diet programs give conflicting messages. The first phase of most diets is often very restrictive: no sugar, no starches ... but the dieter is promised that in the second and third phases she will be able to eat all her desired foods, only in smaller portions. Clinicians for food addicts shake our heads at this advice. If a particular food is your drug, any portion, large or small, will ignite insatiable cravings. In this book, I will explain the physiology of this reaction so that you understand the critical importance of abstinence.

There is good news. Abstaining from problematic foods does not have to be a hardship. Instead, you will experience a freedom from obsession as well as all the negative consequences of addiction. If you think you really are addicted to food, you may never have felt this freedom. That's why I invite you to take the first step: Keep an open mind and read this book. Overcome food addiction now and discover that freedom really does taste great.

THIS BOOK, BITE SIZE:
OUR MESSAGE TO YOU

Christine's Story

November clouds began to drop the first snow of the season as I tossed my book bag over my shoulder and started to walk. I was not happy about the half hour it would take to get home from school, where I was a sophomore. To distract myself, I looked up and caught a snowflake on my tongue.

"Tastes pretty good," I thought to myself, "like a snow cone without the syrup." As I walked, I began to think more about snow cones — lime, cherry, raspberry, grape.

I knew I should not go down this path. I knew that thinking about snow cones, or anything edible, was dangerous for someone carrying thirty extra pounds, especially since I had just started another new diet. I knew from experience that one fleeting image of a cheap carnival confection could be my undoing. I told myself that today would be different, that I would be stronger than the food.

Before I was halfway home, I knew it was hopeless. I had gone from thinking about snow cones to thinking about ice cream with Oreo cookies in it. I started walking faster, so I could raid the refrigerator and the cabinets before my roommates returned.

I started with the M&Ms, stuffing a handful in my mouth, barely chewing them before I swallowed. After scarfing down the rest of the bag, I opened the freezer and grabbed a virgin gallon of vanilla ice cream. It was gone in minutes. Next came the toast with butter and jam, followed by potato chips, salted peanuts with lemonade, peanut butter from the jar, slices of American cheese, a bag of Nestlé's chocolate chips meant for baking.... I didn't stop until I hit oblivion.

Phil's Story

My grandmother died of a massive heart attack at age fifty-two. I can't prove it, but I have come to believe that she really died from untreated food addiction. Of course, my grandmother didn't think of herself that way, nor did her doctor. No one in the medical professional did at that time.

Three decades later, I, like my grandmother, was having trouble with my weight. I kept losing it then immediately putting it back on. One day, after a long day of working too long and a long night of eating too much, I had a heart attack myself. It did not even occur to me that I, my grandmother, or anyone else could become chemically dependent on food.

My food addiction had to get worse before I could address it. A few years later, I had another brush with death that scared me even more. I was sure it was caused by overeating a specific food (wheat), but no matter how hard I tried, no matter what I did, I couldn't stop eating that food for even one day. I felt demoralized and hopeless.

When I shared my experience with a friend who happened to be a recovered alcoholic, he surprised me by telling me, "Phil, you eat like I used to drink."

Those words changed my life.

When an office worker sheepishly polishes off the last cookie from the plate, or a poker player grabs the last slice of pizza from the oversized box, they are not necessarily showing signs that they are addicted to food. There is a difference between simply enjoying food, even to the point of overeating, and having a food addiction. Our brains are wired to enjoy food; it is a primal survival mechanism. We enjoy foods that are high in fat and sugar, because we relate to the immediate energy they provide. Centuries ago, facing a potential famine, these energy-dense "junk foods" might ensure our survival.

In this book, I will explore the science behind the dynamic of food's enticing, mood-altering effects. I will look at why we find food so enjoyable. At the level of the emotional brain, eating, and other activities that encourage survival, such as sex, social interaction, and exercise, are all driven by the same pool of neurochemicals in our brains. These organic molecules, such as dopamine, serotonin, and endorphins (with dopamine as the key carrier), travel specific neural pathways to influence our moods. They give feelings of excitement, comfort, and joy.

Food addiction results when the enjoyment of food has become so euphoric that it dominates our natural impulse to stop when we are full, when the pleasure of eating should be diminished. If the pleasure continues beyond our natural satiation point, something has gone wrong in the hormonal and neurochemical complex that governs our behaviour. Eating with abandon is a biological imperative gone awry. In *Food Junkies* I will explore how this occurs by looking at the mechanics of this frustrating and all-too-common phenomenon.

Today, abnormal eating habits have become a focus of interest, especially in light of the obesity epidemic affecting much of the developed world. Many attempts to understand this phenomenon have been made, principally by dieticians, nutritionists, and eating disorder clinics. Self-help books on how to take off weight are as plentiful as cookbooks. Many experts offer solutions on how to solve our problems with food. Yet no solution has successfully worked over the long term.

Along with many other clinicians in the budding field of food addiction, I believe that by applying the principles of addiction to our destructive eating patterns, we discover the missing piece of the puzzle. I wish to explore the addictive impulse that morphs the normal pleasure of food into what is, for some people, an insatiable and relentless desire. Hot, buttered popcorn becomes a means to settle anxiety; a quart of butterscotch ice cream numbs emotions; a rich chocolate cake provides a burst of euphoria. Food becomes a drug.

Using emerging scientific techniques such as genetic testing, neuroimaging, and neurochemical alterations, scientists and clinicians are finally able to see that some foods have the same qualities as commonly abused drugs. Sugar, for example, triggers the same neurochemistry and neural pathways as cocaine. Sweetened chocolate mimics the effects of alcohol and opiates. Flour modulates moods and anaesthetizes pain just as many drugs do.

Genetic research now suggests that people can be predisposed to becoming alcoholics or drug addicts. This research has found that the same dopamine D2 receptor alterations that are common amongst these subgroups are also found in the obese. Demographic data shows shared familial patterns between alcoholism and obesity. There is also strong demographic evidence indicating that bulimics are more likely than the general population to become alcoholics. In our clinical practices, we have frequently found that alcoholics are more likely to become bulimics once they have stopped drinking.

In a ground-breaking study in the June 2012 issue of the reputable *Journal of American Medical Association* (*JAMA*), researchers report that of the 1,900 bariatric surgery patients surveyed, alcohol abuse increased significantly in the second year after gastric bypass surgery. Sixty percent of these patients insisted that they did not have problems with drinking before the surgery.[1] A more recent study in the *Journal of Surgery for Obesity and Related Diseases* in May 2017 found that approximately one third of participants experienced an uptake in alcohol use or dependence following surgery. I conclude that both conditions, the drinking and the overeating, can be interpreted as different indications of the same addiction. When the person is no longer able to overeat, he or she turns to another means to find intoxication.

As a recovering food addict myself, I am well aware of the daunting physiological force that drives some of us to eat compulsively. I will use my own personal story, as well as numerous stories from my and other clinicians' practices, to put a human face on the current research about food addiction. I will also discuss the solutions that are typically attempted and, finally, the solution that many of us believe is the only one that truly works.

However, many of my readers are more than recovering food addicts. They are also clinicians on the front lines of this baffling and unrecognized condition. I have been an addictions physician for more than twenty years; other voices that I draw upon in this book include long-time counsellors, writers, and educators in the field of food addiction. Many of us have worked with thousands of people who have struggled with food. We have seen many failed attempts to regain control of normal eating, but we have also witnessed a number of remarkable recoveries. I wish to share this information so that you can better understand the complexities of out-of-control eating.

You might wonder whether such a paradigm shift in understanding disordered eating is necessary. Why take the extreme stand of calling the struggle an addiction when that is not a label most people are inclined to accept? Doesn't overeating alone carry enough shame, with its implications of gluttony and greed? Even "foodies," who know that they like food more than the next person — who will say they "love" apple crumble or "couldn't give up their bread" — will deny they have an addiction.

Most people will acknowledge that problems around eating and food exist, and some may even be willing to confess to their own deviant relationship to food. For the extent to which it's now more acceptable to speak out about these disturbing inner demons, we can thank celebrities.

Karen Carpenter was a pop singer with a devoted following in the 1970s. In 1983, the public was stunned when she unexpectedly died of heart failure caused by complications relating to anorexia. Until that time, most people hadn't heard of eating disorders. In her memoir, Gilda Radner wrote of her experience with ovarian cancer and how she struggled with bulimia throughout her comedy career. Radner was a much-loved comic, and, despite her disclosure, her fans continued to adore her.

Actress Kirstie Alley has also lived a cycle of weight loss and gain. In 2008, she had lost about one hundred pounds using the Jenny Craig diet, then gained it back, then lost it again in 2011 using another program: Organic Liaison. Again her weight has returned. This pattern of weight fluctuations has been attributed to a binge-eating disorder. She has been quite candid about her struggles, even chronicling her regimen in her reality show, *Kirstie Alley's Big Life.*

In the early nineties, when biographies of Princess Diana were published reporting on her eating disorder, they opened the door for many to admit to their own bulimic tendencies. Unfortunately, the explanation that I have put forward for these disorders — addiction — carries with it an air of disrepute that adds to the shame already cloaking these kinds of eating issues. Even Oprah Winfrey, who openly admits to a past history of crack abuse, has not declared herself a food addict who has merely shifted her focus from crack to food. Instead, she has positioned herself as the "everywoman" who struggles with her weight by regulating her eating behaviours through diets, personal coaches, and affirmations. Her previous relationship with addiction is in the past, a tasty bit of gossip hidden in her memoir, while she publicly provides her own year-by-year account of her food and weight issues on network television.

Oprah's weight has fluctuated quite dramatically, from 237 pounds in 1992 to 160 pounds in the early 2000s. She has attributed the fluctuations to a thyroid condition and depression, and her success in losing weight to various diets (among them Weight Watchers) as well as personal coaches. She has talked in the past about her relationship with food:

> What I've learned this year is that my weight issue isn't about eating less or working out harder or even about a malfunctioning thyroid. It's about my life being out of balance, with too much work and not enough play, not enough time to calm down. I let the well run dry.
>
> Here's another thing this past year has been trying to teach me: I don't have a weight problem, I have a self-care problem that manifests itself through weight. As my friend Marianne Williamson shared with me, "Your overweight self doesn't stand before you craving food. She's craving love." Falling off the wagon isn't a weight issue; it's a love issue.

It is only recently that food addiction has started to emerge as a self-diagnosis for several celebrities. Singer-songwriter Judy Collins writes compellingly of her food addiction in her 2017 memoir, *Cravings: How I Conquered Food.* She documents how for years she used both alcohol and food in order to be a thin woman as she navigated a successful folk music career. Even more astounding, she writes about her recovery from food addiction using the same techniques we promote in the addiction field: abstinence from the drug (sugar), relapse prevention, and the twelve-step social support network.

Opera singer Deborah Voigt, in *Call Me Debby: True Confessions of a Down to Earth Diva*, similarly writes of her struggles with food addiction. In her 2015 autobiography, she blatantly admits her eating behaviour is addictive when she proclaims, "I was a Poster Child for food addiction." Like so many others after bariatric surgery, Voigt's reliance on alcohol became problematic. She has also found relief from her addictive behaviours through the addictive paradigm of treatment, as well as her faith.

Alas, food addiction has not yet achieved a place in the medical canon. It is odd: Why has behaviour that is compulsive, impulsive, often self-destructive, and even called an addiction in the popular press *still* not been flagged as addictive in the respectable corridors of modern medicine? I believe that this obvious interpretation has been largely rejected for an alternative diagnosis, one that identifies most eating irregularities as primarily some version of an eating disorder.

Indeed, the eating disorder diagnosis, which includes the conditions of anorexia, bulimia, and binge eating disorder, has emerged with an industry surrounding it. Research, medication, and freshly trained clinicians have appeared to help treat the many conditions that have been collected under the rubric of "eating disorders."

While critics in the alternative health communities have demonized particular foods, the focus of medical science has been to look at the pathology of the individual, the behaviour of eating, rather than the addictive content of the food itself. We repeatedly "blame the victim."

That's why I believe that recognizing certain foods and eating behaviours as true addictions is essential. This recognition points to new solutions at a time when the results of the standard ones, such as specialized diets and exercise, have been discouraging. Far too many people, for example, have found that their resolution to diet in the morning dissolves by the end of the day. Even if a diet is successful, most are impossible to maintain beyond a few weeks. The exercise industry is a highly profitable business premised on the illusion that increasing physical expenditure can neutralize bad eating habits. Exercise has tremendous value for physical and mental well-being, but personal trainers are the first to warn overeaters that exercise has minimal efficacy on weight control. Therapy, medications, and surgery also have limited success. Clinicians are puzzled why treatments that work so well in the short term do not, in the majority of cases, result in long-term weight loss or mental stability.

It's time to dispel the shame around food addiction, shine a light into the darkest corners of our psyches, and reveal the private eating and the slippery lies that we tell ourselves and others. I believe that it is imperative to redirect this focus from the individual to the addictive nature of food itself. By including this addiction dimension in our understanding about aberrant food behaviours, we can contribute vital knowledge that has been missed, knowledge that is needed to make a diet work *permanently*.

At the risk of sounding too dramatic, we are running out of time for costly initiatives that will either fail or make little headway. A study by the U.S. Centers for Disease Control and Prevention estimates that by 2030, almost 84 percent of the population will be overweight, and 42 percent will be obese. Even those of us who are not overweight today, or who are just concerned about our intake of junk foods, may have succumbed by then to this deadly epidemic.

My hope is that by shedding light on the addictive nature of food, we will begin to see more effective action aimed at healing this serious sickness, a connection between comfort and food that damages the body, mind, and spirit. Years ago, one infomercial diet coach claimed to be able to help "stop the insanity!" In *Food Junkies*, I will give you a roadmap to help you to eat and feel fully satisfied and in control. Addiction, despite its aura of shame, frustration, and despair, is a beatable foe. You will learn to confront and, ultimately, overcome your compulsion to overeat and step into a brave new world of food serenity.

CHAPTER ONE

EATING, EATING, EATING: WHAT IS THE PROBLEM WITH ME?

It is 1979, late at night. I have been awake for sixteen hours and I'm exhausted and agitated. I pace between my bed and my desk. Should I write my term paper, go out for a run, or recalculate my daily allotment of calories to see if I can afford just one more slab of chocolate? Or just go to sleep, if that's even possible?

I am twenty-three years old and experiencing something I have in common with 25 percent of the female population at Canadian universities — an obsession with weight and food. I am beside myself. My mind is scurrying between one option and another, all in an effort to feel better. I cannot settle. I cannot sit for one minute. Each of my options implies relief, but I know in my gut that none will last beyond even one half hour. Thirty short minutes. How will I ever make it through the night, filled with so many half hours?

If I can just make it to the morning, daytime will bring the relief of distractions, a break from this incessant ruminating. Meanwhile, I feel as if there is a creature inside me, breathing heavily, filling up my insides like a balloon getting bigger and more menacing. It wants to eat ferociously, but if I give it food, even the smallest bit, it will rear up and demand to eat everything in sight. It does not care whether I am full or if I plead with it to stop, my stomach engorged with food, gas, terror. In that moment,

I am just a thin layer of skin containing this monster. It paces and with every slight movement I feel gut-wrenching pain and excruciating anxiety.

I just have to make it to the morning.

Forty years later, having been at this juncture too many times to count, I have found a way to quell the beast. It came only after repeated trial and error and having tried and failed many times to control my urges by creating rules such as eating junk food only on Saturdays, or eating only low-fat, low-calorie items, or eating only in the company of others. I had tried drugging my cravings with alcohol. I tried working non-stop until the cravings passed. Most of the time, though, I just gave in.

Eventually, I found a solution that tamed this creature inside. It was the most effective, yet it was the very last thing I wanted to do, and after each relapse I had to rediscover this truth. Each time, it seemed too ridiculously simple to be true, but at the same time, I thought the solution shouldn't have to be so extreme.

I had to stop eating my favourite foods, the ones that provided immediate relief: the doughnuts, the croissants, the ice cream. Just stop. Whenever I lapsed and tried to revert to what I thought of as the "common sense" notion, that I just needed to learn how to eat properly, I soon slipped back into the same obsessive unmanageability. I would try to have just *one* smallish dessert each night with a nutritious meal. It might take one night, or it might take three weeks of white-knuckling it, but eventually I gave in to the same old pattern of voracious eating. I would start with a slightly bigger dessert the next night; a week later I was eating two desserts a day; the following week it became desserts instead of nutritious meals....

No matter which set of rules I gave myself (only on holidays, only on Saturdays, only low-fat), soon enough the rules dissolved and the obsession was back. So, I finally asked myself, what price was I willing to pay for peace of mind?

I had to see my favourite foods as drugs, despite being aware that most people would think the idea preposterous. But it worked. If I did not drink alcohol, I did not want more. If I did not eat the first cookie, I did not want a second, then a third, then more. The trick was simply not to start eating these trigger foods, because I would just stop, re-start, stop again.

I had spent a lifetime struggling with a solution that had seemed so unpalatable, yet was so successful.

Today, I say that I am an addict. A respectable addict, of course. Not like the desperate addicts who have cashed in their mortgage, the last of their retirement savings, or even cigarette money to get their drug. After all, my drug is cheap, the cheapest of all drugs, and therefore the most pernicious. A bag of day-old doughnuts and a case of root beer cost less than five dollars. And my drug is everywhere I look: in the drive-through gas station's convenience store, in the supermarket, on the lusciously displayed menu of an exclusive restaurant. And my friends, family members, and colleagues are all users. In fact, almost everyone I know abuses food in some way, although if I suggested it they would say, "What, me an addict? No way!"

In those voices I hear my own years of rationalizations. I would tell myself that we all need to eat food, that it is an essential social activity, that I just require better discipline, or that I have had a bad day and deserve a treat. My "common sense" thinking that food cannot be an addiction repeatedly led me straight to yet another relapse, with its secret closet eating, hoarding of food, furtive digging through yesterday's garbage, the bingeing and gorging on pizzas, bagels with cream cheese, bags of chips.

Even at the best of times, when things were going well in my life, I was continually distracted by the thought of food. At lunch, while my friend excitedly told me about her promotion at work, I silently counted the calories of the cheesecake I had just eaten. Could I squeeze in another piece of cake or tactfully get a nibble of hers? I continually forgot, or put off, the resolution that I made the day before never to eat this way again. Whenever I would tell myself this was normal behaviour, it was the addict in me talking. In my heart I knew I was laying the groundwork for the next binge.

All this finally ended fifteen years ago, when I gave up sugar. Today, whenever I tell myself that I can share one small dessert with a dinner companion, I think, *Who am I kidding?*

This is my story. It may not be yours, but I wonder if you can relate to some parts of my tale. Most people can, having felt the lure of some foods that compel them to eat, even against their better judgement. Maybe it's cookies or peanut butter cups. Maybe it's the tease of the ice cream tub in your freezer promising to soothe you at the end of a rough day. Have you ever wondered why you automatically reach for the chips instead of the celery to munch on while watching TV? Or felt guilty that you wanted more cookies and ended up polishing off the bag after planning to eat only two or three? You are not alone. As the food industry is well aware, most people are vulnerable to these temptations.

What can explain this phenomenon? When we consider that more than 60 percent of the population is overweight, it is clear that there is something happening on a grand scale that is affecting a majority of people. Is it addiction? Is it simply poor willpower? Is it something in the food?

Certainly, the quality of the foods that we have been eating has changed over the last thirty years. Much of what we eat contains more sugar, high-fructose corn syrup, and salt than ever before. As I will outline in the next chapters of this book, we are essentially biological creatures motivated by pleasure who, through evolution, now also happen to think. As such, we are wired to desire the more energy-dense foods that will provide us with immediate energy as well as storage for anticipated spells of famine. In short, we are programmed to like sugar and fat. We are at the mercy of our evolutionary heritage even though, in developed countries, the parts of our brain that regulate appetite and hunger have not caught up to the twenty-first century, where famine is no longer the norm. Food is abundant; in fact, it is too readily available, especially artificially created, energy-dense food — junk food.

David Kessler's book *The End of Overeating*, Michael Moss's *Salt, Sugar, Fat: How the Food Giants Hooked Us*, Douglas Lisle's *The Pleasure Trap: Mastering the Hidden Forces That Undermine Health and Happiness*, and more recently Mark Schatzker's *The Dorito Effect* argue that the food industry is deliberately hijacking this universal biological imperative, making foods so tasty, so accurately engineered to target the primal part of our psyche, that few of us can resist them. The food industry is skillful at this; it's their business, and they make good profits from our vulnerabilities.

Societal standards further support eating patterns that are often to our detriment. Think of all the supersize orders and free extras, reassuring us that it is okay to loosen our belts and go for more rather than get up from the table. Eating small amounts seems almost quaint in our era of all-you-can-eat buffets and price deals. At the end of a restaurant meal, the tantalizing dessert that the waiter describes with such great animation tempts us. We may try to resist, but often we give in, shamefacedly and somewhat guiltily. At many work events or family dinners, office co-workers or family members cajole us, even diabetics who are warned by their doctors not to eat sweets, to "have just a taste."

Try not to eat in such social milieus! Saying no to food during celebrations such as those at Christmas or Thanksgiving or on birthdays is especially difficult. How many people have gone on a diet only to find that, despite the success of significant weight loss, they simply cannot maintain their austerity? It is the rare person who will draw unwanted attention to herself by refusing her own birthday cake or the Christmas butter cookies made just for her. The refrain, "Have one! You don't have to be good all the time," follows every dieter. Not surprisingly, it is the rare person who can keep a significant amount of weight off for longer than a year.

Wait a Minute! Does Enjoying Food Mean I Am a Food Addict?

Why is it so hard to say no to savoury foods despite our better judgement? Is it just peer pressure, or do environmental triggers overwhelm our good intentions? More to the point: When does eating food for pleasure become a problem?

We clinicians believe there is something more fundamental than external pressures at work here. The universal human experience of wanting to eat more, especially when delectable foods are on the table, suggests that there is a common dynamic underlying our eating behaviour. For the most part, we have not labelled it an addiction. After all, not everyone who can't resist the lure to eat hyper-palatable foods is a food addict. We are all prone to the lure of food.

What distinguishes addictive behaviour is its extreme nature: the degree to which a person is compelled to eat, is obsessed with eating. Some people are merely tempted, giving in occasionally. Willpower works for them. The sight of a buffet is enough to entrap others, causing them to fill plate after plate of food even after they've stopped enjoying it. Some of us appear to be more susceptible to this seduction than others.

As humans, we all sit somewhere on a continuum, with desire at one end and addiction at the other. Some of us eat for healthy reasons — for nutrition, as part of social interaction and yes, for pleasure. Others eat because they are driven by an insatiable need to eat, regardless of hunger or health — a need that is beyond willpower or common sense. It becomes a need that is disconnected from nutrition, interaction, or pleasure. When an eating behaviour leads to a self-destructive end point, when there is a desire to eat that has no "stop" switch, that trajectory points to the dynamic of addiction.

Let's explore the pleasure of eating, as well as its dangers. It is helpful at the outset to understand why food is so enjoyable in the first place and how that pleasure can overwhelm us and lead to the frustrations that so many dieters experience. When does pleasure become so compelling that it looks like addiction?

CHAPTER TWO

I JUST LIKE TO EAT!
EATING AND OVEREATING

"Hey, if you wore the right clothes and put on makeup, you would look just like *Princess Diana!*"

Janet shyly smiles at the memory of this comment. We are sitting at the round table in her mother's kitchen talking about the trials of dieting. Janet is wearing a pair of blue jeans and a print blouse. She has large square sunglasses on her head and wears a thin silver bracelet on her wrist. She isn't interested in looking like Princess Diana. She isn't a showy person and cares little about current fashions. Even the laser eye surgery she had done years ago was not, she insists, for cosmetic reasons; she wanted to swim in the lake without worrying about her glasses slipping off her nose. Facelifts, Botox, even dyeing her hair are not in the cards for her. Vanity is not her thing.

Janet tells me that she is content with her life. A stressful job and the occasional bouts of nausea that afflict her are the only obstacles she has toward feeling really happy. Although she weighs sixty pounds more than she would like to weigh, she says that her excess weight doesn't affect her happiness very much. "I would be happier if I weighed less," she concedes, "but it is not my main focus."

That's not entirely true, though. Sometimes she wishes that she paid more attention to her weight. When she sees a picture of herself, she feels motivated to diet. When she stands on the scale at her local Weight

Watchers meeting and sees that her weight has crept up another two pounds, she starts to fret. But this lasts for only a couple of days and then she is, again, blissfully unconcerned.

Janet has always been a "chunky" girl and has been on various diets throughout her life. Looking around her parents' kitchen, where she spent her childhood, the wallpaper has been modernized to a light blue pattern, the stove and fridge upgraded, but she can still see herself as a seventeen year old asking her older sister how to diet. They had studied various strategies and she had lost weight with those attempts. "How did I do that?" she asks, recalling those memories of her first diets.

Janet recalls how she always prepared her food ahead of time. She was able to refuse desserts without any distress. She diligently counted and recorded her calories. With each new dietary regimen, she typically lost sixty pounds and kept to her new weight for a few years. But then she would stop following the diet, and as the weight crept back on, her motivation would wane.

At first there were good reasons to get off her diets. She developed gestational diabetes during her first pregnancy. Her doctor insisted that she stop dieting and eat as much as she wanted. Janet smirks, brushing crumbs from the table. "So I ate. I saw it as permission to eat whatever I wanted. I gained all that weight back."

She remembers her husband laughing when he said, "Janet has a new favourite four-letter word: Food!" After her second child, she did not even bother trying to control her weight. Her interest just seemed to fizzle.

Janet joined Weight Watchers in her early forties. She was ready to tackle that annoying sixty pounds once more. Some co-workers from her office agreed to join with her. They all followed the same food plan, shared notes and recipes, and encouraged each other. Janet even convinced her family to follow her meal plan. To her delight, her husband, who was a big man, lost even more weight than she did. Everything was in sync: the family, her friends at work, and her health. It all seemed so simple then. Sighing, she says, "Why can't I do that now?"

Illness derailed her regimen. Janet developed an extreme case of vertigo that still plagues her whenever she is under stress at work. She would get dizzy and sick to her stomach, and sometimes even had to leave work.

Reading or watching television made her feel just as sick, and she would typically end up having to lurch off to bed. "I grew to be afraid of these attacks," she says, the anxiety obvious in her voice. "So I ate." She learned that the only thing making these episodes bearable, even preventable, was food. When she felt an attack coming on, she would reach desperately for something to eat, regardless of whether it was healthy. Anything solid settled her stomach. The bottom line, she tells me, is that she has become more afraid of these attacks than she is about her weight gain. So the weight came back, creeping up even higher than before.

A few years ago, she became alarmed when she saw that her weight had climbed above two hundred pounds, so she returned to Weight Watchers. Shaking her head, she tells me, "I have never been that high."

But Janet discovered what many people who return to dieting find: it seems to get harder each time you go back to it. At first, you're inspired, but soon you're discouraged again. She remembers her first weigh-in after a week of dieting. She had expected to see the typical five-pound fluid loss (both salt and carbs retain water), but instead found she had lost nothing. Not even one pound. "My motivation just deflated then," she says. "It took me one whole month to lose five pounds." Burying her face in her hands, she adds, "All that work for five pounds? Now, I come home and think that I should prepare tomorrow's lunch, but I'm too tired."

The motivator she finally needed? She attributes her most recent weight loss of forty pounds to her son's engagement. Janet has cut down her savoury treats and the late-night snacking and makes sure she walks almost an hour a day. She is determined to fit into a perfect dress for the wedding.

Why Is Eating So Pleasurable?

Enjoying food is not the same thing as being addicted to food. Our brains are wired to enjoy food.[1] It is a primal survival mechanism. In fact, we enjoy foods that are high in fat and sugar for that very reason — they're energy-dense, and they ensure our survival by enticing us to eat more for immediate energy and storage purposes. Even the recovered food addict still enjoys food.

Overeating isn't necessarily a sign of addiction, either. We all enjoy feasting on massive amounts of food. Even if we are full, there are certain times and occasions when we want more. After a satisfying meal, we can usually find room for dessert. This is especially the case when a new food is introduced, because our desire to eat is rekindled by something novel and unexpected. This is why we tend to overeat at buffets. With so many exotic choices, we may fill up on one dish and then suddenly find we have room for yet another tasty tidbit. We leave the buffet with our stomachs bursting, wondering how we could possibly have eaten that much. Our actions are a legacy of our primitive ancestors, who were always aware that food available today might be in short supply tomorrow.

Consuming food is essential to survival, and the pleasure of eating ensures that we do so. Think of it: without the enjoyment, would you bother to buy food (or hunt and gather or grow it), take the time to prepare it, eat it at the risk of becoming bloated, possibly suffering the effects of halitosis, diarrhea, or constipation? When people have colds and are unable to taste and enjoy their food, they often find that they need to "force themselves" to eat. Certain basic human survival needs, like sex and sleep, are related to natural pleasures built into our DNA blueprint; we experience pleasure to ensure we don't ignore our needs. Water is the primary example of this. When you are parched, a cold glass of water is delicious. When you are no longer thirsty, another glass of water has no appeal and can actually be unpleasant. The same is true for food. When we are hungry, the thought of food is pleasurable and the experience of eating even more so. When you are *really* hungry, even a plate of steamed broccoli is immensely enjoyable. When you are full, your desire for the vegetable wanes.

Our hormones and neurochemicals exist as part of a biochemical feedback loop programmed to make sure that this survival strategy occurs.[2, 3] As our stomachs empty, our hunger hormone, ghrelin, is released and tells our brains we are hungry. We begin to feel uncomfortable as the ghrelin increases. The increase in ghrelin levels stimulates the production of the neurochemical dopamine, which makes us start thinking about food. We may think about the approaching dinnertime, about the preparations, about the actual eating experience. Our mouths begin watering, anticipating the pleasure once we finally sit down to eat. The hungrier we are, the more motivated we become. As the motivation intensifies, it can distract us from whatever else we might be doing. The hungrier we get, the harder it becomes to concentrate on reading, driving, conversation....

If we don't eat at this point, hunger actually becomes painful. Thoughts of food become even more prominent, crowding out other thoughts and distracting us from actions that don't lead us to the dinner table. This is the work of insulin, another key hunger hormone. Since sugar is essential to our brain, insulin transports sugar to our brain cells and magnifies hunger to ensure this necessary sugar will be supplied. As insulin rises, we start to feel agitated, eager to start the process of eating. Have you ever noticed that once you've decided to eat, you realize you have a voracious appetite — that, often, you have to restrain yourself from picking at the food before you even get to the table?

In fact, hunger and the desire to eat build from the moment we first start thinking about food. As we anticipate eating, begin imagining the smell of food, and, especially, start to taste the food, insulin levels spike as that hormone prepares to transport the glucose from the food to the brain. This is the premise behind the serving of appetizers. Appetizers stimulate the production of insulin so that by the time we are at the main course, we should be thoroughly enjoying the food necessary for our survival.

When we are full, we no longer desire food, and so the degree of pleasure we derive from eating starts to dip. Our sense of taste diminishes, too, when it is no longer necessary to "fuel up." This curbing of our appetite is also the work of our hunger hormones, which are linked to our endocrine and digestion system. Once our stomach is full of food, our stomach and fat cells release leptin, a hormone that regulates metabolism and body weight and tells us we no longer need to eat. Secreted by adipose (fat) tissue, leptin dampens the potency of the insulin-fuelled dopamine spike that gives us the pleasure of eating. When the reward of eating is diminished, why bother to keep eating? Even though the food may still be pleasurable in theory, without the reward urging us on, we lose interest in it.

Buffets confuse this perfect feedback loop wired into our DNA survival kit. When there are many food choices — those all-you-can-eat restaurant specials, the tables groaning with plates of steaming noodles, roasted meats, candied vegetables, and many varieties of sweets — our dopamine rockets upward, overpowering the leptin intended to halt our eating. Our level of satisfaction with food already eaten is overwhelmed by our desire to explore exciting new territory.

These spikes of desire, followed by curbs that tell us we've had enough, are not specific to food alone; they regulate all pleasures that are intrinsically linked to our survival. We stop drinking water when our thirst is quenched. As for sex, there is only so much a person can have, with nature providing a recuperation period built into our sexual cycles. (The buffet style of sex that exists on porn sites and in magazines has similarly upset the perfect feedback loop inherent in our DNA. The new images artificially spike our dopamine, overruling the signals our bodies produce to tell us that we're satisfied.)

What about social intercourse? No matter how much we may enjoy — indeed, require — social engagement, there is a period of time that we all need to recuperate in solitude. Even the most extreme extrovert will eventually tire of companions who have overstayed their visit. There is a symmetry to our desires and our needs: *We want what we need, and don't want what we don't need.* A perfect ecosystem exists for our primal being, when we are living in a natural environment. The grocery store or restaurant is decidedly not a natural food environment, and that can upset this built-in neurological balance.

Why Do I Eat Too Much?

Overeating is a precautionary defence against an uncertain universe. In part, it reflects the fact that food is not evenly distributed from season to season and across geographical regions. Enjoying food — even too much of it, up to a point — is tied to the natural ebbs and flows of appetite that have evolved to survive in a historically precarious food environment. Disordered eating occurs when our appetites become misaligned with our actual dietary needs. If you continue to want food even when you are not hungry, even when there is a constant source of abundant food around you, something is interfering with your appetite's feedback loop.

What is it?

Certainly, our traditional hunger hormones can be misaligned. For example, abnormal insulin levels, seen in people with diabetes and hyperglycemia, can create a persistent craving for food, regardless of need. A person may have already eaten, but still feel hungry. Recall that as the food from our previous meal is digested and metabolized into its various components, our insulin ensures that blood sugar is escorted to the brain and fat cells. The brain feeds primarily on glucose. When our blood sugar is too low, which happens after hours of not eating, alarm bells start to ring. The hunger gnawing in our stomachs makes us feel agitated, racy, anxious, and eager to eat. The sense of urgency will escalate as our blood sugar drops lower and lower. If we do not eat and get sugar to the brain at some point, our very survival is threatened.

Although hypoglycemia or low blood sugar can be a chronic condition for some people, it occurs naturally whenever a person consumes a lot of sugar. When we indulge in a high-sugar treat like a can of soda, a bag of candy, or a big muffin, insulin spikes to higher-than-normal levels to transport the excess sugar from the bloodstream to the brain and fat cells. An hour later, after the sugar has been transported away, the spike of insulin abates. This is the body doing its job, smoothly and efficiently, and it's a big job to clear away a wallop of sugar flooding the bloodstream. But after the unnatural burst of energy from excessive sugar, we experience an energy crash; as sugar is whisked away into the cells, our system plummets. The result: agitation, ravenous hunger, and extreme anxiety.

People who suffer from hypoglycemia, a condition often thought to be a precursor to diabetes, feel these swings of high and, especially, low blood sugar in a more pronounced manner. It is as if their insulin response is more hypersensitive to sugar, hijacking their physical and mental well-being to focus on food alone. They need to eat right away or else they will feel disabling dizziness, mental fogginess, irritability, and, once again, hunger, hunger, endless hunger. Thrust into a low sugar state, their brains are clamouring for nourishment, usually by way of intense cravings for sugar, since this promises the quickest, most energy-dense fuel.

The medical solution to overeating has largely focused on this hormonal regulator of our appetite. Nutritionists offer diet plans that attempt to curb the excess sugar and stabilize insulin levels. The "diabetic diet" is low in sugar and high in complex carbohydrates (green and brown vegetables) in order to avoid the sugar/insulin spikes.

Unfortunately, keeping our appetite steady is not as simple as following this typical medical diet. Bariatric practitioners who work with obese clients have found that the more a person weighs, the more likely they will become *insulin-resistant*. The insulin receptors in the brain and muscle cells, through overuse from a high-sugar diet, wear out and can no longer manage the task of transporting the necessary sugar needed to keep the body running efficiently. This is what we call Type 2 diabetes. The obese patient becomes permanently fatigued, mentally unfocused, agitated, and, once again, has increased cravings for sugar. Her brain is starved of glucose, even though there are high levels of sugar in her bloodstream.

Science writer Gary Taubes even postulated in his 2010 book *Why We Get Fat and What to Do About It* that receptors in the fat cells become especially efficient at storing fat in the face of excessive sugar loads. Sugar in the blood *must* get removed — ideally to the brain and muscles that use it for energy. If the sugar cannot go to the brain and muscles due to insulin-resistant cells (Type 2 diabetes), it is stored as fat instead. Excessive sugar in the bloodstream will eventually erode the blood vessels, creating blindness, kidney damage, and heart disease. According to Taubes, obesity is a last-ditch effort to prevent the ravages of high blood sugar in a body where insulin is unresponsive. Diabetes (unregulated high blood sugar) and obesity typically coexist as a condition that some called "diabesity." Taubes elaborates on the damage sugar does to our body in his most recent book, *The Case against Sugar*. Here he provocatively suggests that sugar is not only the cause of metabolic syndrome (the common triad of high blood pressure, high cholesterol, and Type 2 diabetes,) but also of arthritis, dementia, and even cancer.

There has been much exploration of other hormonal regulators of appetite, particularly of leptin. A genetic condition of leptin dysregulation, called Prader-Willi syndrome, has been studied for insights into overeating and obesity management.[4] Patients who suffer from this condition have insufficient leptin levels: they are always hungry, regardless of what they have eaten. Not surprisingly, they are very obese and almost always have the coexisting conditions that are part of "metabolic syndrome."

This disease was thought to be extremely rare, but the Foundation for Prader-Willi Research claims that variants of it are under-diagnosed and suggests that there could be many people who suffer from the disease but do not show indicators that are detectable in lab tests. Could there be something faulty about the functioning of leptin in people who overeat?

Overeating and obesity can also occur due to *leptin resistance*.[5] Like insulin resistance, which is a result of the pancreas producing excessive insulin, leptin resistance occurs when too much leptin is produced, creating an overuse syndrome of the leptin receptors. These patients are not suffering from insufficient leptin, as those who have Prader-Willi are; instead, the levels of leptin circulating in their blood are *too high*, so the reward component of eating is suppressed and hunger is never satiated. Like the Prader-Willi patients with insufficient leptin, these people paradoxically feel the effects of leptin insufficiency despite having abnormally high levels of leptin circulating in their blood. Even after eating large quantities of food, they remain hungry.

Scientists have discovered that the more a person weighs, the more likely he will become not only insulin-resistant but also leptin-resistant. This makes sense. Fat cells produce leptin to indicate to the brain that there is plenty of available sugar stored in the fat cells for fuel — no need for more! Increased fat cells lead to increased leptin levels. Increased leptin levels lead to the overuse syndrome of leptin resistance. While increased leptin levels in obesity *should* correlate with higher levels of satisfaction, because of leptin resistance, the opposite occurs.

If obesity causes leptin resistance, leptin may play a larger role in appetite regulation than we imagined. In fact, leptin resistance could be a very common phenomenon. Scientists are discovering that fructose, largely consumed through daily servings of processed foods, can also lead to leptin resistance, regardless of weight.[6]

There has been a drive for a treatment that can overcome leptin resistance. Pharmaceutical companies have attempted to find a "magic bullet" medication to curb abnormal hunger by addressing leptin imbalances. As we will see in Chapter 11, the results, so far, have been disappointing, but valiant efforts are also being made in the nutritional communities.

Changing our diet can make all the difference to avoiding or treating leptin resistance. Two of the most popular of many food plans available are Dr. Jack Kruse's leptin resistance diet, as described in *My Leptin Prescription*,[7] and the diet found in *The Art and Science of Low Carbohydrate Living* by Dr. Stephen Phinney and Dr. Jeff Volek. In both cases, the premise is that a diet high in processed foods has created artificially high leptin levels, so by eating a diet that is low in simple carbohydrates and higher in fat content, leptin levels are subdued and leptin resistance is corrected.[8] This diet will also control sugar and insulin spikes, thus reducing the chance of becoming obese. These clinicians maintain that it isn't fat that makes us fat, but sugar and simple carbohydrates, which are driving up insulin and blunting leptin receptivity.

It has become abundantly clear over the past decade that hormones play a key and complex role in regulating our appetite. The study of these hunger hormones —insulin, ghrelin, and leptin — is promising, yet still elusive. New research and the potential for effective medical intervention have spawned a new discipline of bariatric medicine to complement the bariatric surgical mainstays of gastric bypass and lap-bands. Many new medications and dietary regimens are anticipated in an attempt to redress the hormonal irregularities of obesity.

Is it enough?

Dr Robert Lustig thinks it might be. Working as a pediatric endocrinologist at the University of California, he has treated many obese children who suffer from Type 2 diabetes and other serious conditions more typically seen in an adult population. In an interview with me, Lustig postulated that 20 percent of his patients are "hyper-secreters of insulin" and thus are especially prone to the hormonal effects of carbohydrates. These children are more likely to become insulin resistant and thus obese.

Lustig called these children "carboholics." They are best treated by following a food plan that is low carb as well as fiber rich. Eating "real foods" may not be enough, he warns, recommending they have their carbs drastically reduced in order to keep their weight at a reasonable level. A low-carb diet will also reduce their sugar obsession, since Lustig believes that the desire for sugar is the direct result of hormonal disruption.

These carboholics will benefit from behavioural interventions, such as stress management and exercise. Any behaviour that can lesson anxiety is helpful, since the adrenaline surges that accompany stress also boost insulin. Lustig estimates that a treatment plan that includes a diet of fibre-rich, low-carb foods, more daily exercise at school, and more attention to stress management has turned the trajectory of disease progression to better health in at least 50 percent of his patients.

I believe that, for many, there is an even more powerful dynamic superseding these primal hormonal urges: our neurochemical addiction to food. Some of us eat too much regardless of physical hunger, or pleasure, or stress level. For a food addict, these goals of satiety and safety are beside the point. We just eat because we *want* the food, even if we know we're not hungry. It is all about the overwhelming demand for more, regardless of how much we have just eaten or how full we feel. The satisfaction just cannot meet the want. Our obsession with food is a response to a mental compulsion that is beyond even our powerful hormonal drives to eat. This is what so many of us call food addiction.

CHAPTER THREE

SUGAR MAKES ME HAPPY!

"I was always a chunky child," says Ellen, leading me down a quiet hallway to an empty conference room, away from the lunch hour bustle. We have agreed to meet in the downtown Toronto office where she works as a legal secretary. Ellen is forty-nine, attractive, and heavyset. I thank her for graciously setting aside her lunch hour to discuss her lifelong struggle with weight and dieting. Like so many others, Ellen has many stories of losing weight, gaining weight, losing, and gaining — gaining just a little more with each repetition.

In the conference room there are large windows that showcase a corridor of tall financial buildings outside. We sit at a round black table with eight chairs. There is a whiteboard on one wall and on a credenza sit cups, glasses, and a coffee pot. While sipping coffee, Ellen reassures me that she has already eaten her lunch at her desk.

"I was chubby," she says. "It started when I was four years old."

She has a vague recollection of her mother hovering over her when she was sick, urging her to eat. Even when Ellen's sore and swollen throat made it painful to eat, her mother persisted, fearing her daughter would become malnourished.

As this dynamic continued throughout her childhood, Ellen began gaining weight. By the time she was in elementary school, she was one of the heaviest kids in the class and the other children teased her. Although Ellen's aunt scolded her for eating sweets, her mother discouraged all her attempts to lose weight.

Ellen has a round face and expressive brown eyes. Her hair is stylishly cut and she wears fashionable glasses. Draping a long, black sweater over her purple print dress, she sits with her arms on the table telling me about her life. Today, she lives in a semi-detached townhouse in a suburb of Toronto with her husband and two teenage children. Their home, on a tree-lined street with no sidewalks, is quiet even though it is close to a discount mall just a block away. When her children were younger, they often played in the small park at the end of their street. Ellen says she is happy with her life. She feels especially lucky that her husband has never said anything about her weight over all the years they have been married. It didn't matter whether she was at her lowest weight of 140 pounds or at her maximum of 235, Ned seemed not to notice or care one way or the other. They met when she was quite heavy, so she knows that he loves her regardless of her weight.

Ellen currently weights 217 pounds, which is 60 pounds over her ideal weight. While others might see her as plump or voluptuous, she would be classified as clinically obese by the medical profession. Obesity is defined as a BMI of over 30, and Ellen scores at 38. In fact, Ellen would actually be classified as morbidly obese and thus runs a higher than average risk of suffering hypertension and arthritis at some point in her life. She has already been diagnosed with diabetes, a by-product of her obesity, which she is attempting to control through diet.

Ellen's relationship with her mother has always been fraught with tension; she crosses her arms over her chest as she tells me about it. Her mother was frequently ill: she had diabetes, heart issues, even breast cancer in her later years. She was always obsessed with her poor health. Numerous hospitalizations meant that the children often stayed with other families. Ellen was much closer to her father, always a "daddy's girl."

Ellen could not understand why her mother was so upset whenever she tried to lose weight. Her mother was overweight as well and had tried many diets herself, so why not see Ellen as a comrade in the weight wars? Instead, her mother baked regularly and would be irritated if Ellen refused her homemade offerings. Most of the time, it just seemed easier to accept rather than face the guilt or hostility. It didn't help, Ellen admits, that she has always had a sweet tooth.

Ellen remembers sneaking down into the basement when she was ten years old and stealthily eating food late into the night. She would cram food into her mouth, moving from one shelf of treats to another. "There were always cakes and cookies, and lots of them," she recalls. "I liked the sweets, not the chips and nuts that other people ate." Although her mother encouraged her to eat these treats, Ellen had a hunch that bingeing was not acceptable behaviour.

When she got married, this secret bingeing continued. In public, she made a point of eating normal portions of what she thought of as "good" food. She ate properly at dinners and with friends, but privately, when no one was home, or late at night when her family was sleeping, she would slip downstairs and eat whatever sweet food she could find in the kitchen. There was always something in her house, since both her son and husband loved baked goods as much as she did.

When I asked her about her relationship with food, she laughed and said: "I love food. I don't eat to live but I live to eat. Food is my friend." I was struck by how quickly she answered, without having to search for the right words.

When I asked Janet (from the previous chapter) the same question, she was puzzled: "Relationship to food, what do you mean?"

Janet clearly had a relatively detached relationship to food. Ellen intuitively knew that she depended on food as an aid to survive in the world, much like addicts feel about their drugs. They often refer to their drug as their lover or best friend.

When Ellen was fourteen, she went on her first "official" diet, despite her mother's objections. Her girlfriends had been talking about the Scarsdale Diet, which was popular at the time, and she wanted to fit in. She doesn't remember many details about that diet, but she can recall eating slices of ham and grapefruit at her school desk while others around her ate pizza and drank cola. When she lost weight, Ellen was pleased with her success and promptly stopped the diet. To her surprise and dismay, she slowly gained back all the weight she had lost.

Since then, Ellen has been on so many diets they've become a blur in her mind. It was always the same: she would lose weight, stop the diet, and then regain the weight. Ellen is not alone in this experience. Estimates vary: from one-third to three-quarters of the population is on a diet on any given day. One U.K. study of over 1,400 subjects showed that British women spend an average of six months a year on a diet and more than 20 percent are on a permanent diet. The researchers averaged out their data and concluded that thirty-one years of a woman's lifetime are spent on a diet.[1]

Confirming what Ellen discovered after trying each new diet, a European poll found that amongst six hundred people scattered across seven European countries, more than three-quarters of respondents were on, or had just been on, a diet. Most had been unable to avoid regaining weight. In many cases, dieters actually regain MORE weight, leading to the quip: "How to gain weight? Go on a diet!" Estimates suggest that only somewhere between 1 and 10 percent of dieters keep off their weight after one year.[2] Ellen's experience is the heartbreaking story of so many — after an initial success, there is a slow decline into disappointment and shame.

Ellen continues to tell me about the diets that she can remember. There was the cabbage soup diet, memorable because it did not work at all, even while others purportedly watched the pounds melt off. Another diet had her eating only five hundred calories a day: cottage cheese, eggs, and very limited carbs (some melba toast was allowed). Rolling her eyes, she told me that she ate so much cottage cheese that, to this day, she cannot eat it without feeling sick.

She found that, while some of these diets were successful, none were sustainable. After a year of eating food from the Nutrisystem diet — a concoction of powders and shrink-wrapped portions — she came to hate the food plan. Deprived and cranky, she yearned to eat "normal" foods again. Weight Watchers worked for her, although only if, she admits rue-fully, she worked very hard at it.

Today, she says reflectively, she has identified the pattern that so many people fall into over a lifetime of dieting. At first, she would adhere to the rules of each diet, preparing her foods and, in the case of Weight Watchers, counting her food points, documenting her weight, and going to the weekly meetings. She would lose thirty pounds, but then, despite the success of her weight loss, she would gradually drift away from the rules, the groups, the weekly weigh-ins. Inevitably, her weight would slowly return.

Five years ago, when Ellen was diagnosed with diabetes, she was very reluctant to go on medication. But when her doctor told her she could reverse her condition with diet and weight loss, she was motivated to try once again. She signed up at a medical weight-loss clinic in her office building.

At the outset, the physician diagnosed her as having a binge-eating disorder. She was floored. There was a name for her condition? A diagnosis for her eating behaviour? She found this comforting, since she'd long ago realized she was different from other people, who seemed to be able to control their eating. However, she only needed to look at her family to see the differences. Her husband was oblivious to what he ate and, to her annoyance, remained thin no matter how much junk food he consumed. On nights in, when they snuggled together to watch TV on the couch, he often offered her his tub of ice cream. "I'm on a diet," she would remind him. He typically gave her a sly smile and coaxed her, "But just one small scoop won't hurt, will it?"

He simply did not understand her struggle.

Nor did her daughter. A lean and athletic seventeen-year-old, she kept to a strict meal plan without any qualms about it. She didn't seem to battle the same feelings of deprivation and resentment that Ellen felt whenever she had to refuse some mouth-watering item. Food just didn't seem to be that important to her daughter.

The medical clinic proposed a meal plan that consisted of eating a specific proportion of proteins, fats, carbs, and fruit. The plan was similar to the one offered by Weight Watchers, but with one important difference: she was not allowed to eat *any* sugar. She was taught behaviour-modification techniques to identify and manage the food triggers that made her want to keep eating even after she was full. This was the first time that she had heard a doctor declare that she was using her food as if it were a drug. This rang true to her. "Yes," she concluded to herself, "I *am* using food like a drug."

This time, Ellen lost weight and felt invigorated and healthy. For the first time in her life, she did not crave sugar. She leaned toward me, splaying her hands. Something new had happened to her, she said. She found that she had entered a "zone" where she could refuse any food offered to her. Intuitively, she knew, without understanding why, that if she even had the taste of sugar, she would be thrown out of this zone. That would be the end of her diet. So, she told me, "I did not touch sugar. I can't have just one cookie. I was afraid to eat a cough drop."

Ellen is an all-or-nothing type of person.

Then one day the inevitable happened. She was at a birthday party and the hostess offered her a sliver of birthday cake. Ellen smiled weakly, protesting that she was on a diet. Her friend chuckled and teased her. "Not even one little bite?"

Ellen sighs, remembering the fateful moment. "I couldn't get around this. I had to eat it. How could I say no?"

She took a nibble from the cake on the paper plate, already knowing she would finish the piece. She resolved to restart her diet the next day. Her motivation was still high after having the experience of feeling great for months. She hoped that memory would carry her over this risky bump.

Before she knew it, she went off the rails. "I went straight back to eating the wrong things at the wrong times," she says. "Sweets, pretzels, fruits. What happened to my motivation to stay on the diet?"

Ellen was shocked at the suddenness and power of the relapse. She had really thought that the onset of diabetes would have frightened her into staying on the diet. She also thought that if she did fall off the wagon, the memory of how good she'd been feeling would make it simple to return to her diet. She struggles to explain what happened. "When I lost the focus, I was not in the zone anymore. Then everything felt like deprivation. I could not imagine *not* eating sugar. It just seemed impossible." Today, Ellen is clear that she uses food like a drug. "Food is a stress reliever," she explains. "I eat when I get home. It helps to ground me, relax me."

She tries to eat healthy foods to compensate: crackers and hummus or fruit instead of cookies and chips. When she is upset, however, she still reaches for sugar.

"Sugar," she says, shrugging, "makes me happy."

I explain to Ellen the concept of food addiction. To a food addict, eating even just a little bit of sugar, or any other trigger food, will set up the phenomenon of cravings that leave her wanting more. Just one cookie is enough to act as a trigger; like a lit match to kindling, it inflames a highly volatile reward pathway. It's just waiting to be set ablaze, an inferno that consumes willpower and makes it impossible to rationally moderate portions after that first taste.

Ellen nods, agreeing that food does this to her, just as that one sliver of birthday cake did. I see the relief she feels in knowing that there is a term to explain this lack of focus, this derailing of motivation. It is more than a failing of willpower. It seemed to capture her experience more accurately than the binge disorder diagnosis, which described her eating behaviour, but not what actually triggers her binges.

Really? Food Addiction?

Is everyone who eats too much a food addict? No. But the question of where to draw the line between behaviour that merely indicates the enjoyment of food at one end of the spectrum, and behaviour that is symptomatic of someone suffering the persistent and annoying cravings spurred by addiction at the other end, is a difficult one to answer. While it is true that almost everyone can be tempted to eat too much of the wrong things, at least some of the time, I contend that some people, like Ellen, experience that temptation so often that it compromises their physical and mental health.

The next chapter will investigate why food tastes so good and why it makes you feel better — why it can soothe or even make you giddy at times. Understanding the basic neurobiology of pleasure, and how particular foods bolster this pleasure, will explain why it is so difficult to say no to the offer of a sugary, fatty confection. Food addiction is a disorder related to this fundamental level of desire. What makes some people simply unable to control their diet, despite the best of intentions and determination? Answering this question is the goal of this book, a journey toward understanding the very nature of food addiction.

CHAPTER FOUR

SO, WHAT EXACTLY IS FOOD ADDICTION?

Louise's Story

Picture this: a marching band of ants, complete with conductor, playing drums and singing:

Food, food, food, food …

That is what is in my head all day.

I wake up and my first thought is, "What shall I do for breakfast?" Should I drive through Tim's and get a muffin? Yogurt? Doughnut? Twenty Timbits? Full breakfast at the local eatery? Maybe just a coffee and then I'll get a mega-muffin from the bakery.

Food, food, food …

It's around 10 a.m., time for a smoke break … umm, I wonder what we're doing for lunch. Swiss Chalet? Chinese? McDonald's? What do I feel like?

Food, food, food …

It's 11 a.m., I can't wait for lunch …

Food, food, food …

It's 11:30 a.m., I wonder if I should go have a smoke now and meet the gang at the restaurant after I'm done?

Food, food, food, food …

Here we are at the restaurant. What to have? I can always say I'm not going to have time for dinner so they don't think I'm a pig. I can be healthy — yah, sure!

Food, food, food …

It's 2:45 p.m. now and my stomach's rumbling. Perhaps a bag of chips, a chocolate bar, or some ice cream? If I buy for everyone in the office I won't feel so guilty.

Food, food, food …

Wow, 4:00 p.m. already. I'll call Joe and see if he wants to grab a bite. Indian? Chinese? Local pub? Maybe I'll just go home and order in. Dinner for four from Chinese-A-Go-Go? Family pack from Swiss Chalet (with two desserts of course)?

Food, food, food …

Driving home, 5:30 p.m. Better stop on the way and get some supplies for the night. Will it be salty or sweet?

Food, food, food …

I'm home, it's around 7:30 p.m. What shall I munch on? Popcorn, chips, a loaf of bread?

Food, food, food, food …

Sitting by myself at 10 p.m., lonely, tired, depressed, stressed. I'm hungry again. How about a chocolate bar?

Food, food, food …

Having a good day? Having a bad day? Friends aren't around tonight? Feeling down and depressed? Feeling up and excited? It doesn't matter how I feel, food makes it more extreme. Happier, sadder, worse, better. Or, if I do it right, I can eat so much I'll just pass out; no time to feel whatever it is I'm feeling. Oblivion at last.

No, I'm not going to overeat. I will start a new diet regimen tomorrow, first thing in the morning. Fruit and yogurt for breakfast, no snacking, salad for lunch, proper balanced dinner, no TV snacks. That's it. I'm tired of feeling physically ill. You'll see, I can do it. Tomorrow! I promise.

But when tomorrow comes, I start overeating, yet again.

———————

Enjoying food is not the same as being addicted to food. Our brains are wired to enjoy food; as we have seen, it is a primal survival mechanism. In fact, we all enjoy foods that are high in both fat and sugar for that very reason. They're energy-dense and ensure our survival by making us want to eat more for immediate energy and storage purposes. Whether you're a normal eater, an overeater, an undereater, or even a recovered food addict, everyone enjoys food.

Disordered eating occurs when the natural ebbs and flows associated with the pleasure of eating are scrambled. In the last chapter, we touched on the hormonal reasons that can explain disordered eating. Hormones such as insulin and ghrelin, our traditional "hunger hormones," can be misaligned. When we become hypoglycemic, with our blood sugar level plunging to dangerously low levels, we become agitated, almost frantic, in our need for food. An imbalance of the ghrelin and leptin hormones that govern our food satiety can also leave us feeling perpetually hungry, no matter how much we have eaten. I believe that the neurochemistry of addiction trumps even these most powerful and primitive drives.

The Neurobiology of Pleasure

How can something as seemingly benign as a sliver of birthday cake lead to the total destruction of body, mind, and spirit? How can a person wake up in the morning and think about nothing other than food from the time she opens her eyes until she falls asleep late at night, in a puddle of ice cream and cookie crumbs?

When we choose to eat rather than go to see a friend or hang out with the kids, when we keep eating despite feeling bloated and uncomfortably full, something is driving us, something a lot more powerful than the rational part of our brain that whispers, "You'll feel better if you don't." Saint Matthew got it when he said, "The spirit is willing but the flesh is weak."

There are powers at work in the human body that can override the best of intentions.

It's just the body doing its job.

As a result of our biology, we are motivated to fulfill essential tasks of survival, such as eating, procreating, and sleeping; accomplishing these tasks is motivated through a reward-seeking mechanism built into our brain. This mechanism is in a deep, primitive part of the brain made up of complex neural processes called the *limbic system* (found in the paleomammalian brain).[1] The limbic system, is a complex cluster of nerve cells comprised of the ventral tegmental area and the nucleus accumbens. It is located beneath the cerebral cortex and the frontal lobe, and directs our moods, motivations, and instinctual behaviours toward survival-enhancing functions. The specific neurochemicals that are involved in these processes — the "happy" ones that create pleasure — are *serotonin, dopamine,* and *endorphin.*[2]

Serotonin makes us feel calm, satisfied, and content. We are experiencing an abundance of this chemical when we feel grateful and content about our circumstances. It is also the neurochemical that propels the feeling we commonly have when, for example, we are socializing in a meaningful way, feeling as if we belong to a group. We need it in order to sleep. It is the neurochemical that produces the warm fuzzy feeling that might make us think, *I have everything I want and need.*

Dopamine gives us a natural, excited high, the feeling associated with the expectation of pleasure. Dopamine sparks the eagerness we feel on a first date and the allure we get from reading a really good book. It's also responsible for the thrill we feel as we anxiously await the lottery ticket numbers to be read over the airwaves, and the satisfaction we experience after achieving a long-sought-after goal. Dopamine is our natural "curiosity" neurochemical. Counteracting complacency, it stimulates us to meet new people, find new jobs, and generally seek new experiences in life. It is the neurochemical that gives us enthusiasm as we feel anticipation.

The endorphins are our natural pain relievers. When we are hurt, endorphins flood our brain and body so that we are numbed to pain, mental or physical. The pain-relieving effects of endorphins explain why a person can still limp after rupturing a tendon or can still cope despite experiencing a calamitous event. Sometimes the person exalts in the crisis, feeling a sense of mastery of the situation and none of the anxiety sure to follow when the mishap is resolved. Later, though, the emotional or physical pain will come in full force as the endorphins subside.

Endorphins also give us the energy to get out of dangerous circumstances. A mother who is able to lift concrete blocks in order to save her infant during a bombing raid can do so because of endorphins. The many people attracted to crisis situations, extreme sports, body mutilation (cutting, burning), and, of course, exercise are seeking an endorphin boost. The so-called "runner's high" is a natural endorphin rush. We only feel pain the morning *after* the workout.

The rewards that these neurochemicals provide are essential to survival. Eating, sex, sleep, and so on must be pleasurable to ensure we do these things that keep us alive. The reward must be robust enough to motivate us even through painful or frightening circumstances, like fatigue, cold weather, or danger from threatening predators roaming outside our lair. Yet, while the reward must be strong enough to motivate, the reward circuitry must also "sense" when to let up on the rewards so that we're not so attracted to pleasurable activities that they will do us harm.

For example, too much of serotonin's easy contentment can actually de-motivate a person. This often occurs when someone is stabilized on an anti-depressant. *Why do more if I am content with what I already have?* the patient sometimes wonders, no longer wanting to return to work after a period of short-term disability has run out. Unrestrained dopamine can lead a person to risk-taking activities, such as extreme sports, or to addictions to such things as gambling or Internet porn. An over-reliance on endorphins can lead an individual to seek out stressful practices, such as physical fighting, or self-mutilating behaviour, such as cutting or slashing.

We achieve serenity when we find an ideal balance of these neurochemicals. We thrive best when we have a good deal of serotonin, as when we are in familiar and friendly circumstances. And we need to have enough dopamine to be stimulated, with the occasional introduction of a novel circumstance, such as a new person, food, or book. It is my experience that we do best when 80 percent of our feelings relate to safety and social ease (linked to serotonin), and 20 percent of our feelings relate to novel experiences (which spike our dopamine), just to spice things up and keep us from getting bored. Too much stimulation, however, disturbs our general sense of well-being, which is premised on feeling safe and unruffled. When we get anxious, we seek out stabilizing routines to ground us.

We also need to have access to plenty of endorphins, to cope with the discomfort of stress or injury. Overall happiness seems to be the level at which these neurochemicals are balanced appropriately to each individual's temperament.

All too commonly, however, problems occur with these neurological mechanisms of motivation. Rewards can be too diluted to have any effect. Depression, for example, occurs when rewards are so dulled that they are barely discernible; a person does not wish to eat, have sex, or socialize. Why bother if there is not enough return for the effort involved? If there is no satisfaction in doing something, the depressed person may not see the point of doing anything, even getting out of bed.

On the other side of the reward continuum lies the potential for addiction. Human nature, imperfect as it can be, often leaves us wanting far more than reality can deliver. But there is always a limit to how good a reward can get. The peak of a sexual experience subsides within minutes; the exquisite taste of a piece of good chocolate eventually wanes.

Dr. Robert Lustig put it well in his interview with me last November 2017: "You can think of reward as having a bell-shape curve. There's a sweet spot in the middle. Anywhere else on the curve and you play with fire."

When we want more than life can realistically deliver, we are expected to curb our desires. In order to do so, we learn skills of emotional regulation, skills that are essential for negotiating the balance between "have" and "want." Each one of us has experienced examples of unbridled enthusiasm that fall flat, leaving behind dashed hopes, disillusionment, even despair. Most of us work through these experiences, learning to tailor our expectations to match what is realistically possible.

Crossing the Line: From Pleasure to Addiction

Perhaps more than anyone else, addicts experience the dilemma of wanting more than is realistically possible. They want more and more and more; it's as though their on-off switch has no "off." Whatever the person gets is never enough. "I can't get no satisfaction" is the plaintive cry of the addict. Nothing in reality can match the need, since the need is artificially boosted.

This artificial need — or, in the case of food cravings, "false hunger" — can be the result of an imbalance due to insufficient serotonin: the "nothing is good enough" exasperation that many despondent people experience. No matter how good the experiences, without the necessary serotonin to actually create the feeling of satisfaction, the person is left unmoved. Or it can be due to an excess of dopamine, whereby the person may not even know what it is he wants, just that he *wants*… something, anything. We call this experience of wanting the "phenomenon of craving." Alcohol, addictive drugs, gambling, *and* food can all fire up the reward pathway to heights that our evolutionary brain cannot possibly achieve naturally. These, and intense behaviours that provide excessive gratification or anticipation, like shopping or Internet games, can hijack the limbic system, that primitive and crucial part of our brain. They give a big payload of "happy neurochemicals" to the nucleus accumbens, which results in the artificially high load of expectation that is the euphoria of intoxication.

Drugs that boost serotonin levels are primarily hallucinogens or psychedelics, such as LSD, mescaline, ketamine, magic mushrooms, and PCP. Drugs that hijack the dopamine surge, maximizing it to unstoppable heights, are cocaine, crack, amphetamines, Ecstasy, and even nicotine. Behaviours such as gambling and shopping, where anticipation of the result plays a big role, can also produce a dopamine rush. Drugs that mimic endorphins are in the opiate family and are used clinically to minimize physical or emotional pain: codeine, morphine, oxycodone, methadone, and hydrocodone. Alcohol provides access to an abundance of all three neurochemicals; which is why alcohol intoxication can give the drinker an enhanced effect of all three experiences: safety and sociability, excitement, and a numbed, pain-free state of mind. Small wonder it is so universally popular.

Clinical experience has indicated that if these substances are introduced into the brain at a faster pace, gratification is heightened. A person who drinks on an empty stomach gets drunk more quickly, since the absorption of alcohol is not competing with food. If a person injects a substance rather than ingests it, the transit time to the brain is shorter and the drug experience is that much more euphoric. Snorting or smoking a substance produces the most potent high and the fastest road to tolerance and addiction. Immediate gratification is extremely compelling. Ogden Nash had it right when he quipped, "Candy is dandy but liquor is quicker."[3]

We see evidence of this with opiate medications, typically used to treat severe or long-term pain. Even though the doses are often high and the drugs are potentially addictive, when patients take these medications orally (especially in a slow-release format that gives a steady level of the medicine over hours), the opportunity for addiction is minimized. But, when a user chews the pills — thus destroying the slow-release mechanism — or snorts or injects the drug, it has a powerful and almost instantaneous effect on the brain, increasing the likelihood that the patient will become addicted.

This hijacking process can be explained by neuroscience. We know there is a system of neural structures in the brain that controls behaviour by creating pleasurable effects. This is known as the "reward system." The source of addiction — whether alcohol, a drug, the act of gambling, a sexual encounter, or certain foods — causes the nucleus accumbens to receive the pleasure-inducing neurotransmitter, dopamine. The intensity and speed of a drug's entry to the brain provides the immediate gratification, or "quick fix," that is at the core of addiction. This is not the result of natural causes; it has been artificially created via the production process of the drug itself.

Let's look at alcohol as an example. When animals in the wild nibble on fermented grapes, they feel so lazy and sleepy that they stop eating long before they would become drunk. The alcohol content of unprocessed natural sugars (fermented grapes, honey, soggy rye) is at most 5 percent.[4]

But when the alcohol content of fermented grapes (or grain, in the case of spirits) has been enhanced into the potent alcohol we're familiar with (13 percent in the case of wine, 40 percent in the case of whiskey and other liquors), the brain's ability to moderate consumption is bypassed.

The same is true with cocaine. There are only so many coca leaves that an animal can chew before it grows weary of chewing. However, the cocaine that creates rampant addiction has been chemically extracted from coca leaves. The intense, near-instantaneous euphoria it creates in this form makes users want to snort or inject, regardless of weariness or any other inhibition to consuming the drug.

Finally, food: The fibrous stalk that protects the sucrose of sugar cane, or the thick bark protecting the sap in a maple tree, limits the amount of sugar that a primate can ingest. But if one harvests and removes the sugar from the sugar cane or transforms the maple tree's sap into syrup (or removes the honeycomb from a beehive to extract the honey), the product is one of the primary raw materials contributing to food addiction. It's so easy to drop sugar cubes into coffee or pour maple syrup on ice cream, yet doing so sets up an extraneous "unnatural" process, which allows us to circumvent the consequences that would otherwise curb our consumption. We are able to experience an artificial high from the refined product that is far more powerful than what the natural version would otherwise allow us.

So the big payoff of addiction comes about when the reward is unrestrained by the limitation of what life can deliver through natural means. Our reward circuitry becomes highly sensitized, anticipating the promise of a greater and more substantial prize. It's the dangling carrot leading the galloping horse out of the corral, unable to stop even when its muscles are straining with fatigue. Addiction, with its promise of the big payoff, motivates us to act even in the face of extremely dangerous consequences, even when the promise is impossible to attain. Addiction is the land of never-ending want.

No one knows precisely when a person will cross the line and begin to choose artificial over natural rewards, but we do know that artificial substances work because, as shown above, *they are more intense and more concentrated than natural rewards.* There are many things in life that induce pleasure, but what matters is the potency of the stimulant. For example, sex gives a dopamine surge of about two hundred units, while cocaine, in comparison, releases four hundred units. It's generally accepted that our brains can handle between one hundred and three hundred units before addiction kicks in.[5]

It's as if our brain were designed to run on diesel and suddenly we're giving it rocket fuel. Our grey matter has not evolved quickly enough to handle these surges, to efficiently temper these super-charged rewards. We are not yet able to negotiate what is helpful under extreme circumstances (such as a feast after a time of starvation) and what is not helpful on a regular basis (overeating without cause).

So, when exposed to unnaturally high surges of the happy neurochemicals — serotonin, dopamine, and endorphins — the brain tries to adapt. From the first intake of any drug, the brain attempts to adjust to the novel circumstances by reducing ("down-regulating," in scientific terminology) the receptor sites in the limbic system to match the sudden onslaught. Within a matter of days or weeks, a person develops a tolerance to these surges and no longer feels their impact as powerfully. A "new normal" has been created.

The memory of that new normal has now been cemented into the neurological wiring of the reward center in the limbic system. Not only do addicts crave the heightened experience, they actually *need* it just to feel normal. But the new normal will soon feel insufficient, since the nature of addiction is always to want something more, bigger, better. Addicts seek the big payoff — that unforgettably glorious high they experienced the first time they tried the substance — but their brains' efficiency at adapting thwarts them. The brain, it turns out, is skilled at creating a "new" new (another way of saying "tolerance"), so more of the drug (or behaviour) is required to amp up the volume of that elusive pleasurable feeling. Each time, the brain adjusts again, and the cycle continues until the addicts find themselves in dangerous territory. In the addiction field, we call this "chasing the dragon."

If replicating the first high is not attainable, neither is stopping the drug use. Addicts quickly discover that when they stop their drug of choice, they feel distress. Abruptly cutting off that excess flow of neurochemicals leads to a crash that far exceeds any normal experience of depletion. For any of us, a day of excitement, such as a graduation or a wedding, often leaves us exhausted the next day; we feel we are "running on empty" and need to retreat for a few days to replenish ourselves. The depletion that occurs in the addictive cycle mirrors the artificially induced overabundance of neurochemicals. As high as a person goes, the crash is equally low.

The result is a person who is physically, mentally, and spiritually bankrupt. Depression, anxiety, insomnia, and a plethora of other symptoms of withdrawal follow. Most of us can handle the lethargy we feel the morning after a big event, but the enormity of despair that follows an addict's high would tax even the most strong-willed amongst us. Clinicians call this neurochemical bankruptcy "post-acute withdrawal syndrome" (PAWS); addicts call it a hangover, cold turkey, or just feeling absolutely, hellishly wretched.

At this point, the stress response kicks in, making a bad situation abysmally worse. The drug user now transitions from using their substance for the euphoria effect, what psychologists call positive reinforcement, to using the drug simply to avoid painful withdrawal. This is called negative reinforcement. The brain interprets the pain inherent in withdrawal as danger and sparks our primal survival response to combat the risk ahead. Adrenalin and anxiety surge, acting as powerful motivators to keep using, despite the grave consequences. The "short-term gain" of immediate relief from acute withdrawal is far more important than the "long-time pain" of ongoing destructive drug use.

Reason and emotional regulation rest in the frontal lobe, where our executive functions — thinking, reasoning, and compassion — attempt to moderate our primal drives and instincts. With acute addiction and withdrawal, it becomes impossible to rein in the ramped-up desire for euphoria or its counterpart, the fear of cold turkey. Soon, the streetcar of desire has careened off the rails. Willpower, never a consistent or reliable ally, even at the best of times, is collateral damage.

This is why addicts are powerless over their addiction. While they may be desperate to get clean — jobs, families, homes may hang in the balance — when their reward and stress circuitry is hijacked they usually feel utterly powerless, unable to control their urges. Even when in recovery, cravings and urges will always occur. For most, it is impossible to neutralize triggers such as old friends and familiar haunts, or visual cues such as seeing people drinking or using needles, in person, in movies, on TV, or in advertising. Sometimes cravings occur without the provocation of a trigger; sometimes they are neurologically imprinted. For individuals with this problem, their powerful wants remain, acting on an emotional and instinctual level, even if the rational part of their brains tries to resist.

So, Is Addiction a Disease, a Choice, or Both?

Perhaps the most heated debate in the addiction field is whether addiction is a disease or a choice. Typically a physician who relies on neurochemical and brain imaging data will declare that addiction is a disease just like any other mental disorder, such as depression or anxiety. If levels of hormones or neurochemistry are changed, and this difference causes disruption of the body's or brain's homeostasis to the point of impairment, the condition is considered a disease. We could push the point further. Addiction can even be viewed as a physical disease like diabetes or hypothyroidism. These conditions have much in common: blunted receptor sites, misaligned hormones, neurochemicals which, if untreated, cause disruption and impairment of normal daily activities.

The anti-disease, choice spokespersons tend to come from the ranks of psychologists who rely on the operant conditioning model of behaviour. Addiction is *learned behaviour* and can be understood by applying a formula: stimulus (trigger) leads to response (using). A person who has been abused and neglected in childhood, and who has not learned adaptive strategies for coping with psychic pain, may eventually find the lure of drug use compelling. Changing the formula by nullifying the rewards of drug use with medication or by increasing the value of sobriety through tangible rewards, such as cash vouchers and social support networks, can stop addictive behaviour in its tracks.

The oft-quoted phrase from Johann Hardi's 2015 Ted talk, *Everything You Think You Know about Addiction Is Wrong*, that "the opposite of addiction is not sobriety. The opposite of addiction is connection" illustrates this point. Hardi claims that what we really want, whenever we engage in healthy or unhealthy behaviours, is to connect with others. So providing strong connection can *and does* alter addiction. Witness the tremendous power of twelve-step programs, where the high value placed on fellowship has saved the lives of many addicts.

As a clinician, I make the diagnosis of disease whenever the motivation to act a particular way pushes a person beyond the intended survival endpoint (e.g., food enjoyment and satiety) into the realm of injury. A person who eats to the point of illness, or works too hard, or has obtrusive sexual urges, basically wants more pleasure than normal life can possibly provide. If motivation (spurred by dopamine) is hijacked, heightened, exponentiated by a substance, the disease is evident.

While people may choose to pick up a drink or a drug, they cannot choose the neurological wiring that drives their ramped-up desires and motivations. They may stop themselves from picking up their fork, but they will still *want* to eat. We call this ongoing desire without its corresponding behaviour being a "dry drunk."

Choice, a frontal lobe mechanism, is time-limited and tenuous. Addiction counsellors have discovered that "frontal lobe fatigue" seems to occur in about twenty minutes under the fire of multiple temptations. After fighting against their artificially spiked desire (dopamine), people ultimately succumb. Or they will be angry, irritable, and discontent. "Give that man a drink!" "I will start the diet again tomorrow!" This is the call of a typical dry drunk.

Addiction is both a disease *and* a choice, to be visualized on a continuum of desire. A person can *start* with the ability to choose using drugs when the desire hits. But eventually, because addiction is chronic and progressive, ongoing use will tug the person toward the disease end of the spectrum, where obsession and unmanageability of drug use are foremost. At the end of the line, choice is eventually trumped by the more primitive diseased limbic system, which cannot stop wanting.

The discussion of whether addiction is a disease or a choice is highly relevant in the field of food addiction. A central theme of this book is that both clinicians and the general public are resistant to acknowledging food addiction as a disease. Problematic overeating is interpreted as a mismanagement of choice. But, why not envision the level to which food is addictive as a marker on the continuum of desire? Depending on where a person rests on the continuum, they either still have choice or they eat nonstop, despite heroic efforts to restrain themselves.

Allowing this range of response to addictive foods allows us to develop a range of effective treatments. It enables us to tailor our treatment to the degree to which we still have choice (using controlled portions of trigger foods, cognitive therapy, mindfulness), including interventions that will serve the hopelessly addicted (recommending residential sugar detox).

There is no one treatment that works for all. In fact, treatment parameters often need to change even in the lifetime of one person. What worked ten years ago may no longer work today. Some people can moderate their consumption of trigger foods for a while, only to find out years later that they have a growing list of foods from which they must now abstain. Addiction is progressive and complex, and not so simple as to be either a disease or a choice.

Food: The Slower Picker-Upper

Awareness of the addictive nature of food is on the rise, but there is not yet widespread recognition that food can lead to full-scale addiction as powerful as those involving alcohol or cocaine. One reason is that, unlike other addictive substances, food, unless consumed quickly and in large quantities, does not give the same kind of rapid feeling of comfort. It takes thirty minutes of eating before a person settles into that warm, numb place. It offers less a *sudden shifting* of reality than a *gradual easing-into* a new place. Alcoholics often vividly remember their first drunk, whereas most food addicts will not remember their first sugar buzz. It is a "slower picker-upper" in contrast to drugs or alcohol.

It often takes food addicts years to develop the sort of full-blown addiction that has them hugging the toilet or calling in sick the next morning. It's a gradual, but insidious, progression from one lump of sugar in coffee to four, or from a few bites of candy to a supersize bag. Food addiction easily slips under the radar: obesity, diabetes, high blood pressure, and depression are all consequences of food addiction, but they are usually identified by their individual symptoms rather than by the underlying cause. The digestion of food is slow and the effect on the brain prolonged; it's not until food is eaten quickly and in enormous quantities that the surge of happy neurochemicals mimics the euphoria provided by a drinking bout or a line of cocaine. If food addicts could smoke or inject sugar, food addiction would be on the same playing field for researchers as cocaine or heroin.

This understanding of the pharmacokinetics of addiction (pharmacokinetics is the study of the path of a drug once administered) has misled even researchers who study the addictive nature of food. Neuroscientist Dr. David Linden and other researchers halfheartedly call fats and sugars "faintly addictive substances," thus failing to grasp the essence of why something is addictive.[6] It is the *intensity* of the neuro-chemical surge and the *immediacy* of the substance's transit to the brain, more than the nature of the substance itself, that propels addiction. The quicker the fix, the faster the addictive process. Cocaine is, in a sense, the equivalent of a big bag of sugar ingested at higher speed.

If eating could trigger the same level of neurochemicals as cocaine, we would get the same euphoric effect and drive to consume more. And we do. Food addicts on a tear consume large quantities in a short time. To be clear: achieving this involves not just overeating — consuming a bowl of potato chips or plate of cookies — but wolfing down the entire bag or box and then going out and buying three more for the night. Under these conditions, food is just as virulently addictive as alcohol and drugs.

Like other addicts, those addicted to food have preferences for the kind of euphoria they seek. The drinker may choose between the lazy, slow high of beer that is drunk throughout the day versus the hard, acceler-ated punch of a three-martini lunch. Some food addicts may favour soft creamy foods, like ice cream, that provide comfort. Warm milk, pasta, potatoes, bananas, and turkey provide bursts of serotonin, making them feel warm, soothed, and sleepy.

Others may prefer harder, crunchier fare — foods high in sugar or white starch, for example, which boost dopamine, providing bursts of startling energy. Rats, given amphetamines for one week, later developed the same speedy hyperactivity from sugar intake alone, highlighting the similar dopamine spike from both substances.[7]

Chocolate, dairy products, spices, and, yes, even sugar, produce the anesthetic effect of endorphins. When was the last time you were in pain and found that chocolate made you feel better? Parents frequently discover that sugar is an effective analgesic for infants, working as well as acetamin-ophen. Scientists have shown that medications used to treat alcohol and opioid cravings can also be used to moderate food cravings. The fact that Naltrexone (ReVia), an endorphin blocker, can work to dampen sugar highs points to the opioid-like nature of sugar.[8] Experimental evidence has also shown that rats will exhibit the same withdrawal pattern from a week-long sugar binge — twitching, pacing, and sniffing — as they do during opiate withdrawal. A similar study by Princeton psychologist Dr. Bartley Hoebel found that when rats exhibited addictive behaviour, changes were found in both their endorphin and dopamine receptors.[9]

Small wonder that well-meaning members of Alcoholics Anonymous will suggest that a newly sober member eat a candy to fend off cravings.[10]

The simple substitution of one addictive substance for another often calms the agony of withdrawal. In his fascinating book *Wheat Belly*, William Davis bluntly draws a parallel between popular agricultural products, like wheat and sugar cane, and alcohol: "Beer is just liquid bread, or bread is just solid beer; rum is just liquid sugar, or sugar is just solid rum." Fermentation and distillation merely alter each product's constituents. The net effect is similar: a boost of the three happy neurochemicals to the nucleus accumbens (the reward pathway), resulting in a feeling of warmth and excitement and a dulling of the senses. Given this, it is no surprise that patients who have had bariatric surgery such as lap-band surgery (and who are, thus, unable to return to their old eating habits) have a much higher risk of developing alcoholism.

Science Catches Up: Food Addiction Exists

The last ten years have yielded exciting research to corroborate our understanding of neurochemical addiction to food. Bart Hoebel and his team are among the first of many now exploring, and *proving*, the connections. Even formerly skeptical scientists have begun probing further, not content to stop with sugar. They have tested artificial sweeteners on their rats to measure merely the *anticipation* of sugar. To their surprise, they found that rats *preferred* saccharine to sugar. Many food addicts agree with this startling discovery, admitting that it is only when they stopped their diet soda drinks that their cravings for sugar abated.

Paul Kenny and Paul Johnson at the Scripps Research Institute in Jupiter, Florida, conducted the *crème de la crème* of animal studies and food addiction. These researchers found that by overfeeding rats in a laboratory setting, they could literally turn the rodents into food addicts.[11] "These studies," wrote Pat Harman in a review of the Scripps study for *Childhood Obesity News*, "show that over-consumption of high-calorie food can trigger an addiction response in the brain." Ongoing research by Pedro Rada and Nicole Avena shows similar findings: when sugar and fat is introduced into rat chow, the experimental rats find the resulting mixture highly compelling.[12]

It is on this premise that Dr. Avena and John Talbotts's book *Why Diets Fail (Because You Are Addicted to Sugar)* is based. They posit, as I do, that in order to stop eating the processed food that contributes to weight gain, we must stop eating the key ingredient saturating that food — sugar — which drives the addiction. In her newest book, *Hedonic Eating: How the Pleasure of Food Affects Our Brains and Behaviour*, Dr. Avena summarizes the science regarding these concerns about sugar, as well as other key factors (impact of dieting and manipulations of the food industry) that explain our unhealthy attachment to food.

Not content to let the naysayers argue that we should not extrapolate from animals to humans, another crop of scientists has taken a different approach. Using sophisticated neuroimaging technology, such as functional MRIs and SPECT (single-photon emission computed tomography), these researchers have been able to measure cerebral blood flow and brain activity patterns of people in the throes of their addictions.[13] These studies have been instrumental in expanding our understanding of what goes on in a brain affected by alcohol, drugs, or food. What neuroimagists have discovered in users of these substances is that when the limbic system, the hub of all pleasure, is flooded with dopamine, it literally "lights up" with activity.

Chief among the imaging studies is one led by Dr. Gene-Jack Wang at the Brookhaven National Laboratory Institute.[14] Wang and his colleagues used PET (Positron Emission Scans) to compare dopamine activity in ten obese and ten normal-weight subjects. They found that the overweight individuals had fewer dopamine receptors than their normal-weight counterparts. These individuals need to eat differently (more food, foods with higher sugar or fat content) to get the same satisfaction that a leaner person gets.

Genetic research has also added to the scientific evidence for food addiction. We have known for some time that there is a genetic predisposition to alcoholism: in a small percentage of cases, we can find evidence of dopamine receptor alterations[15] that can distinguish a social drinker from an alcoholic. There appears to be a similar (perhaps the same) genetic indicator for a predisposition to becoming obese.[16] This points to the possibility that a person who is predisposed to alcoholism may also be predisposed to food addiction and obesity.

Carolyn Davis, a professor of kinesiology in York University's Faculty of Health in Toronto, examined genetic markers in both obese individuals and people with binge eating disorder (BED). What she and her colleagues found was that BED subjects had significantly higher scores on a self-report measure of what her team called "hedonic eating." In her summary of the study's findings, Davis and her colleagues suggested that BED is a biologically based subtype of obesity that may be activated by a genetic predisposition. Davis concluded that genetic studies "provide significant support for the general working hypothesis that dopamine system genes play an important role in feeding behaviour and obesity."[17]

This link is reinforced by the finding that there is strong demographic evidence that bulimics and people suffering from binge eating disorders are more likely than the general population to become alcoholics.[18]

Food addiction exists. Although the science that supports it is still in its infancy, it may be useful to remind the critical reader that addiction research in general, whether for alcohol, cocaine, Ecstasy, or opiates, is at a similar early stage. Clinicians are drawing upon research that is still based on animal experiments and sophisticated radiological scans, and they mainly rely on hands-on "gut" experience — both their own and those of their colleagues — to inform their diagnoses and treatment decisions. Once food addiction is recognized in the clinical realm, we will have a similar wealth of data to inform us.

But we are getting ahead of ourselves. First we need to know how to spot a food addict. What does a food addict look like? How do you know if *you* are a food addict?

CHAPTER FIVE

ARE YOU A FOOD ADDICT?

- Have you ever wanted to stop eating and found you just couldn't?
- Do you think about food or your weight constantly?
- Do you find yourself attempting one diet or food plan after another, with no lasting success?
- Do you binge and then "get rid of the binge" through vomiting, exercise, laxatives, or other forms of purging?
- Do you eat differently in private than you do in front of other people?
- Do you eat to escape from your feelings?
- Do you eat when you're not hungry?
- Have you ever discarded food, only to retrieve and eat it later?
- Do you fast or severely restrict your food intake?
- Have you ever stolen other people's food?
- Have you ever hidden food to make sure you have "enough"?
- Do you obsessively calculate the calories you've burned against the calories you've eaten?
- Do you frequently feel guilty or ashamed about what you've eaten?
- Do you feel hopeless about your relationship with food?

If you have answered yes to more than three of these questions, you are most likely a food addict.[1] And if you can relate to the following conversation, overheard between an addiction counsellor and a client trying to kick the bingeing habit, you might just qualify:

> **Client:** Yesterday I ate all day long. I started with breakfast — big three-cheese omelette, home fries, six pieces of toast. Then I had two raisin bagels with cream cheese, six chocolate-glazed doughnuts with a pint of milk and something else — I can't even remember what, I was in such a fog. I do remember that for lunch I wanted to eat something "normal," so I went to a buffet and ate a salad loaded with cheese and cold cuts and tons of blue-cheese dressing and bacon bits. In the afternoon I had five or six candy bars, a bag of corn chips, and a couple granola bars. I went home then and passed out. But then I got up and went out for pizza.
>
> **Counsellor:** When do you think you lost control?
>
> **Client:** The minute I got out of bed! I told myself that I wasn't going to eat sugar — sugar really sets me off — but it was like I was two people in one body or like somebody else was driving and I was the car. No matter what I said to myself, I still picked up the food. I had one voice telling me to go ahead and one voice telling me not to.

Sound familiar?

Am I Really a Food Addict? How Can I Tell?

How can we know if we are really addicted to food? *Addiction* is a term that's used a lot these days. People claim to be addicted to everything from romance novels to cars. They feel guilty when they enjoy something just a little *too* much. When it comes to food addiction, the misunderstanding is epidemic. Office workers whose weight would be considered normal sheepishly say they are addicted to cookies when they take the last Oreo from the break room. Women who simply enjoy the occasional plate of pasta turn to their partners and say with a sigh, "I wish I weren't so addicted to spaghetti." Are they clinically *addicted*?

My esteemed colleague Philip Werdell, a gentle, soft-spoken man in his seventies, is part of a group of professionals dedicated to raising the visibility and understanding of food as an addictive substance. He says, "If it looks like addiction and responds to treatment like an addiction, then why not call it an addiction?"

How can we tell? Until now, scientists and clinicians alike have been reluctant to acknowledge that food addiction even exists. Yes, abnormal eating behaviours have been identified throughout history, but there has long been a resistance to labelling them an addiction. Challenge Werdell about it and he grows militant. "The position that there is no scientific evidence supporting the existence of food addiction, and there-fore there are no food addicts, flies in the face of research gathered over the last fifteen years," he says. "There are well-designed animal exper-iments, detailed brain imaging studies, and more than three thousand peer-reviewed writings.[2] Such blanket, and often unsupported, criticism is just plain anti-science and anti-intellectual, much like the debunking of global warming."

As far as he is concerned: If it looks like a duck, walks like a duck, and quacks like a duck, it's a duck.

The duck has been quacking for quite some time, probably as long as food has existed. But a surge of overeating over the past thirty years (during which time the public has indulged in the supersizing trend in restaurant meals, the larger soda bottles, etc.) has resulted from the industrial processed-food complex, which has exponentially increased the reward potency of food.[3] The one benefit, though, has been a grad-ual softening of the public's reluctance to see chronic overeating as a true addiction. But we are impatient with the pace of change. Until all clinicians acknowledge this diagnosis, the identification and treatment of food addiction remains hampered.

A Brief History of Food Addiction

In 1960, the twelve-step fellowship Overeaters Anonymous was founded by an overweight woman named Rozanne after recognizing that her overeating was similar to the uncontrollable gambling addiction of a friend. After attending a meeting of Gamblers Anonymous, she was cited by OA historians as saying, "Our compulsions were not the same. They were obsessed with gambling and money, and I thought of nothing but overeating and food. Still, inside we were the same."

In 1975, William Dufty wrote the bestseller *Sugar Blues* in which he made the case that sugar is an addictive substance that can be compared to drugs such as opium, morphine, and heroin. He blamed the white stuff for a wide array of physical ailments, from acne to mental illness. He had no peer-reviewed literature, no double-blind studies, no MRIs or PET scans to back up his claims, only his own history and that of other believers who knew how they felt while eating sugar: unhealthy and out of control. Dufty and his cohort called the sellers of sugary foods "pushers."

In 1981, a twenty-nine-year-old woman who was unable to stop bingeing on food approached a well-respected alcohol rehabilitation facility to ask for help. This woman, who wishes to remain anonymous, described her behaviour to the intake team. The head of the facility, shaking his head in surprise, remarked, "That sure sounds like alcoholic behaviour to me." She was admitted on an experimental basis, since the team had never before treated anyone addicted to food. Her counsellor wisely advised her to think about food whenever she heard the word alcohol.

In 1986, a psychiatric hospital called Glenbeigh, in Tampa, Florida, opened a companion unit to its drug and alcohol rehab centre that was to be devoted entirely to treating food addicts. Before closing in the early nineties, Glenbeigh managed to establish itself as *the* place to go if you couldn't stop eating. Patients described the horrors of their addiction in vivid detail. Their adventures included stealing food, getting stopped by the police while driving and eating, taking food out of the trash, "blacking out" after overeating, and eating well beyond the pain of a distended stomach only to then resume the binge after the pain subsided. Collectively, they had gained and lost hundreds of thousands of pounds and spent enormous amounts of money on food, diet drugs, and weight loss schemes. Many had thought about, or attempted, suicide.

Four years later, Dr. Frank Minirth and Dr. Paul Meier of the Minirth-Meier Clinics published a book called *Love Hunger: Recovery from Food Addiction*, which chronicled their development of a method to treat food dependency alongside their comprehensive, spiritually based counselling practice.[4]

In 1993, mental health counsellor Kay Sheppard published a revised version of her signature work, *Food Addiction: The Body Knows.* Sheppard drew from her experience working with food addicts and did not mince words. "Food addiction is a chronic, progressive and ultimately fatal disease," she wrote. "It is chronic because the condition never goes away, progressive because the symptoms always get worse over time, and fatal because those who persist in the disease will die an early death due to its complications."

Then, in 1996, Judi Hollis became one of the first professionals to publish academic findings about food addiction, doing so in her book, *Fat Is a Family Affair: How Food Obsessions Affect Relationships.*[5] Hollis, an addictions counsellor, noticed that her own problems with food were quite similar to her clients' problems with drugs and alcohol. She convinced William Rader, a former director of the chemical dependency program offered by the U.S. Navy, that many of the obese and those with eating disorder symptoms needed to be treated as if they were addicted to food. This led to the establishment of a network of Rader Clinics throughout the United States.[6] Her book became required reading for their patients.

In 2005, Nora D. Volkow, director of the Maryland-based National Institute on Drug Abuse (NIDA), began to connect the dots between food abuse and other addictions.[7] As an addictions physician, she was instrumental in having food classified with the plethora of other addictions that American physicians were responsible for treating. Writing in the scientific journal *Nature Neuroscience,* Volkow highlighted studies linking dopamine levels in compulsive overeaters and cocaine addicts. Among other findings, she cited brain study research that recorded dopamine increases in humans who simply *looked* at images of food. Volkow wrote, "In some obese individuals, the loss of control and compulsive food taking behaviour share characteristics with the compulsive drug intake observed in drug-addicted subjects." She put food addiction on the medical map.

Four years later, Dr. David A. Kessler, former commissioner of the U.S. Food and Drug Administration, published *The End of Overeating: Taking Control of the Insatiable North American Appetite.* Echoing Volkow, Kessler shared his own experiential evidence for the addictive nature of food as well as some of the science current at that time, explaining the brain chemistry behind food cravings and compulsive eating. Kessler stopped short of calling the phenomenon an addiction, opting instead to use the term "conditioned hypereating."

Also following the lead of Dr. Volkow and NIDA, in 2011 the American Society of Addiction Medicine (ASAM) redefined the nature of addiction itself. No longer a matter of poor choice or poor emotional control, the ASAM officially defined food addiction as a brain disorder. Certainly, will-power plays a role in curbing the behaviours endemic to addiction, but it is the smallest factor in the successful management of addiction. "At its core, addiction isn't just a social problem or a moral problem or a criminal problem," says Dr. Michael Miller, past-president of ASAM, who oversaw the development of the new definition. This disease "is about brains, not drugs. It's about underlying neurology."

The ASAM has taken great strides in proclaiming that addiction can involve pretty much *any* substance or behaviour: the classic culprits are alcohol, drugs, gambling, or sex, but the Internet and food are also candidates for what are now called "process" addictions. If the object of one's compulsion fits certain criteria (see the ABCDE of addiction[8]), it qualifies as an addiction. The organization is also insistent that, like cardiovascular disease, diabetes, or depression, addiction must be treated as a chronic condition; it has to be treated, managed, and monitored over a lifetime. People who are addicted must learn the tools to keep their urges in check and apply those tools on a continuous basis.

The ASAM also warns clinicians that addiction is progressive if left untreated. Any food addict will agree, aware that where one bursting bag of popcorn might have been sufficient in the early days, now neither the bag nor the extra candies nor the supersize pop will satisfy. As discussed in the preceding chapter, the neurochemical excess leads to measurable physiological changes in the brain, which in turn leads to a rising tolerance and an ever-greater consumption of food, as well as withdrawal symptoms similar to those of any other addiction once the bingeing has stopped.

How Do We Diagnose Food Addiction?

As the medical profession has come to accept food addiction as a real condition, there has developed a need for a method of *diagnosing* the condition — a way of determining whether a person has an eating disorder, has an addiction, or is just not motivated enough to stop after the first bite.

So far, there is no lab test to determine if a person has *any* addiction, let alone a food addiction. There are no radiological procedures to guide clinicians, although innovations in neurological radiology are transforming modern research. Over the last five years alone, due to neuroimaging innovations such as functional MRIs and SPECT scans, scientists have published many illustrations that strongly suggest a link between our brain's propensity toward addiction and food.

Within the next decade, we can expect that physicians will find external markers to determine addiction in the same way we expect to diagnose clinical depression or ADHD.

Today, however, we base our diagnosis of addiction mainly on questions and observations — we look for the specific attributes that coexist with addiction. The questionnaire I presented at the outset of this chapter is part of the toolkit, which several twelve-step food addiction programs use to determine if someone is a food addict. If you answered yes to just a few of the questions, it is likely you are a food addict.

But because, so far, food addiction lacks an official diagnosis, scientists and clinicians usually apply the American Psychiatric Association's *Diagnostic and Statistical Manual of Mental Disorders*

(*DSM-5*) criteria for general addiction (referring to the category called substance use disorder) to food to help them make a diagnosis. The *DSM-5* is a world-renowned compendium of categories that document all recognized mental disorders. It provides a specific set of criteria for each psychiatric condition so that a diagnosis can be made and universally understood.

The *DSM-5*, the most recent update, was released in 2013, but despite significant lobbying efforts, it did not address food addiction. It did, however, introduce binge eating disorder (BED).[9] So far, this inclusion of BED has not had any impact on the diagnosis or treatment of food addiction, although there are currently attempts to define a subset of BED sufferers as food addicted. If food addiction can get official recognition, if only through this "back door" of becoming a subset of BED, services for food addiction treatment may become available for insurance coverage.

Clinicians in the field have slowly started to use the *DSM-5* criteria for addiction to diagnose food addiction, but most of the tools being used today to diagnose and study food addiction were formulated using the *DSM-IV-TR*. These tools are in the process of being revised and scientifically validated to reflect the changes found in the new version of the *DSM*. In any case, the *DSM-5* modifications do not alter the criteria to make a diagnosis of addiction; instead, they combine the *DSM-IV-TR* categories of substance abuse and substance dependence into a single disorder measured on a continuum from mild to severe.

Many of the *DSM* criteria for substance use disorder overlap with those of other eating disorders, such as bulimia or binge eating disorder. This makes the new art of food addiction diagnosis especially confusing: it is possible that a patient can be a food addict *and also have an eating disorder*. Most of us in the field believe that many people who have been diagnosed with a binge eating disorder, for example, are actually food addicts. For this reason, the next chapter will look at other types of eating disorders that can overlap with food addictions and result in misdiagnoses.

The DSM

The *DSM-IV-TR* and *DSM-5* provide guidelines for clinicians to follow when making a psychiatric diagnosis. As noted above, the *DSM-5* maintains the same criteria for diagnosing addiction as did the *DSM-IV-TR*. A patient has a substance-use dependency if he or she has developed distress from at least three of the following at any time within a twelve-month period (distress from all six would be classified as severe addiction, according to the *DSM-5*):

- Patient has developed tolerance or withdrawal symptoms.
- Patient has frequently taken more substances than planned.
- Patient has taken excessive time acquiring, using, or recovering from the effects of the substance.
- Patient continues to use the substance despite difficulties.
- Patient has given up work, social, or family activities if they interfere with using.
- Patient has made multiple attempts to cut down on use of the substance.

Keeping these guidelines in mind, clinicians observe the typical behaviours that their addicted patient displays to make the diagnosis. We can see the patterns that exist for food addicts by looking more closely at the typical behaviours of people who abuse food.

The single most important feature leading physicians to suspect addiction is that patients experience cravings and obsessions surrounding their drug of choice. For the food addict, cravings are typically focused on foods that are high in sugar and fat: the muffin for breakfast, the latte loaded with sugar and cream at lunchtime, the apple cruller on the way home from work. Anyone can look forward to snacks when she is feeling hungry, but a food addict is thinking about her favourite foods all day, whenever her mind is not otherwise occupied. She may even be thinking about her next snack before she has finished the last one. These cravings can be just as insidious and powerful as an alcoholic's cravings for another drink.

Cravings for food can even be triggered by quantity alone. Large amounts of food, even healthy foods, can overwhelm the body's hormonal regulation and satiation signals. The more you eat, paradoxically, the more you want. I once met an addict who would munch through three large bags of carrots a day, eating so many that her skin turned an orange hue. She did this simply to have the experience of putting something in her mouth, savouring the chewing, crunching, and swallowing.

Withdrawal symptoms constitute another major criterion of addiction. Recovering from a food "hangover" can last for days. Critics often use this criterion as their proof that food addiction does not exist: they insist that there is no measurable physical withdrawal from a food binge — that is, no DTs, seizures, goose bumps, or diarrhea. I have often scratched my head at their reluctance to recognize the signs of withdrawal. I wonder if they have actually asked a person who has just binged on five thousand calories of sugar and fat how they feel the morning after. I have seen the withdrawal symptoms: not seizures, true, but snappy moods, insomnia, tremors, nausea, aching muscles, and a mental fog that can be as dramatic as any alcoholic hangover.

Substance abuse upends the normal activities of daily life. Work and social events are almost always impacted by ongoing drug or alcohol abuse. An alcoholic may not be able to get through the day without surreptitious swigs of vodka, thus jeopardizing his job. Similarly, a food addict can spend a good portion of his day thinking obsessively about food. He will typically plot his day around meals and snack times, often using food as a motivator to get him over the next hump. He might be getting through the workday by promising himself a spicy cheese pizza and tub of caramel ice cream at the end of the night. Food becomes the reward, the payoff for a hard day at the office.

Some food addicts may be grazers, constantly eating small quantities, such as a handful of peanuts, a bag of jelly beans, a bagel, or a banana, all to help them quell distressing feelings that would otherwise interfere with their lives. How is this different from slipping into the bathroom for a quick puff on a cigarette? Food addicts can, alternatively, be binge eaters who consume large quantities of food in order to soothe their anxieties or to numb their emotional pain.

Obsessing about food, painful as it may be, usefully distracts from other, more painful, emotions.

Planning a menu of scrumptious trigger foods, preparing the "stage" — selecting the activity that would allow for endless eating (like a Netflix binge or playing cards) and picking the foodie companions that will also overeat as much as the addict — can be tremendously time-consuming, but is part of the pleasurable feelings addicts experience long before the actual eating occurs. Calorie-counting and excessive exercising after a binge can consume hours. The depression and shame that typically follow can also take days to dissipate and often herald the next binge. Any behaviour that encroaches on our day so thoroughly that it impairs other activities and takes up prolonged mental space is a red flag indicating addiction.

Habitual binge eaters will often find that they are too uncomfortable to follow through with their commitments after a binge. Who wants to socialize when suffering from a gaseous and bloated abdomen? Like alcoholics, food addicts often forgo seeing their friends and end up isolating themselves. Asking someone out for dinner or even coffee may invite shame, rejection, or reprisal, and of course it takes time away from their favourite activity. Why bother with social activities, the food addict thinks, when he can just turn on the tube and eat potato chips instead?

Einstein's remark that insanity can be defined as continuing to do the same thing repeatedly while expecting a different outcome is often cited in the field of addiction treatment. Repeating the same self-destructive behaviour, despite negative consequences, in hopes of a positive outcome is a hallmark symptom of addiction. This is what we call denial. It provides the foundation of distorted thought processes which is popularly known as "stinking thinking."

Make no mistake: food addicts, like other addicts, intuitively know that they are engaging in self-destructive behaviour. But they do not want to dwell on this. The food addict knows she is obese; she has probably been warned by her physician to lose weight too many times to remember. Her hypertension, diabetes, and sleep apnea are all clear consequences of her food intake. These are monstrous anxieties that a food addict has to manage on a regular basis.

How can she live with this ongoing anguish? The food addict's system of denial becomes ever more complex and defensive as the addiction progresses. She reaches for the most bizarre rationalizations to quell her anxieties:

- The diabetes isn't that bad yet.
- I can get away with this binge one last time.
- I may as well go all out since I blew it today.
- The diet starts tomorrow, definitely.

These are typical examples of the delusional process of "stinking thinking." The more knowledge a well-meaning professional gives to the food addict, the greater the addict's need for denial. Meeting with her doctor usually does not inspire the food addict to change her eating behaviour, but rather makes her feel discouraged, defensive, and even more confused.

The mainstay of addiction is the inability to stop using, despite repeated efforts. How many dieters do you know who have attempted to stop or cut back and been successful over the long term? The dieter starts off with good intentions to cut back her portions of bread and pasta, but finds that she eventually returns to eating these foods. Or worse, she begins eating even more. She tries to have just one cookie but finds that, inevitably, she eats the whole bag. The food addict simply cannot stop — not for long. The desire for the trigger foods overwhelms her willpower.

The Yale Food Addiction Scale

The above discussion highlights the ease of applying *DSM-IV-TR* criteria to abnormal food behaviours. Some scientists have attempted to develop a scale that is specific to food. We in the field need a common tool to share scientific knowledge and clinical experience. The peer-approved Yale Food Addiction Scale (YFAS), released in 2009, is one such tool.[10] (Although a newer Yale Scale based on the *DSM-5* is currently under study, the first Yale appears to be more widely preferred.)

The YFAS marks the first step toward professional credibility of this disease. You can see how these questions capture many of the observations that clinicians have made about their patients who struggle with overeating. I anticipate that this is the tool that doctors of the near future will be using to diagnose their patients.[11]

Below is the shortened version of this scale, the YFAS. If you answer yes to three or more of the following criteria, you could be suffering from a clinical addiction to food.

1. I find that when I start eating certain foods, I end up eating much more than I had planned.
2. Not eating certain types of food or cutting down on certain types of food is something I worry about.
3. I spend a lot of time feeling sluggish or lethargic from overeating.
4. There have been times when I consumed certain foods so often or in such large quantities that I spent time dealing with negative feelings from overeating instead of working, spending time with my family or friends, or engaging in other important activities or recreational activities I enjoy.
5. I kept consuming the same types of food or the same amount of food even though I was having emotional and/or physical problems.
6. Over time, I have found that I need to eat more and more to get the feeling I want, such as reduced negative emotions or increased pleasure.
7. I have had withdrawal symptoms when I cut down or stopped eating certain foods. (Please do NOT include withdrawal symptoms caused by cutting down on caffeinated beverages such as soda pop, coffee, tea, energy drinks, etc.) For example: developing physical symptoms, feeling agitated, or feeling anxious.
8. My behaviour with respect to food and eating causes significant distress.

9. I experience significant problems in my ability to function effectively (daily routine, job/school, social activities, family activities, health difficulties) because of food and eating.

These tools are a godsend to those of us working in the food addiction field. Finally, here is a way to tease out the tangle of disordered eating behaviours. Until now, clinicians and food addicts alike have been confused: when is overeating a binge or an addiction? When is it poor willpower? Is an anorexic or a bulimic a food addict, or can they be both? The confusion is endemic, and is likely to persist for some time given that there is an overlap of symptoms and conditions as well the residual reluctance of mainstream practitioners to acknowledge that the beast exists even when it is staring them in the face. The following chapter will illustrate this particular mess.

CHAPTER SIX

THE FOOD FIGHTS: ADDICTION OR EATING DISORDER?

The 1990s was the decade of the food fights. Professionals began arguing about the underlying problems associated with chronic obesity. Was it the result of an eating disorder or an addiction to food? Was there such a thing as a normal eater who just ate too much? For years, leading nutritionists had argued that the entire problem of obesity could be attributed to an imbalance of "calories in and calories out."[1] People simply ate too much and did not burn off the necessary calories to keep their weight stable. To solve the problem, they needed to be educated about food choices and encouraged to exercise.

Members of the various professions working with people who struggled with their eating issues argued that the underlying problems for the obese were deeper social-psychological traumas, which led people on a trajectory toward an emotional dependency on food. When confronted with the proposition that food could have a chemical lure more powerful than the emotional, clinicians argued that the concept of food addiction was "without convincing empirical support," and turned, instead, to the research on eating disorders to probe the nature of and treatment for their obese patients.[2]

Yet, as early as 1960, Overeaters Anonymous had produced evidence that a twelve-step program that dealt with food as something addictive, in the same way that alcohol, drugs, or gambling can be, could help compulsive eaters by recommending *abstinence* from certain foods. According to this thinking, obesity is the product of a neurochemical disease; calories are not the issue, nor is insufficient exercise. Joining this camp were the self-declared food addicts, who passionately disagreed with the established perspective that obesity was caused by poor willpower. Noted spokespeople, such as Kay Sheppard, Anne Katherine, and Joan Ifland, wrote self-help books that made the case that people who could neither diet successfully nor control their eating were actually *addicted* to food.[3]

So, a disagreement had developed: Was abnormal eating the result of an addiction, an eating disorder, or just plain gluttony? For decades, at the annual conference of the International Association of Eating Disorder Professionals, panels of experts debated the topic: *Is There Food Addiction? Pro or Con?* True believers debated the issue at length, with neither side successful at convincing their opponents.[4]

We even found the same debate within Overeaters Anonymous. For more than a decade, the central theme of each OA World Service Business Conference has been whether compulsive overeating is the result of psychosocial-emotional disturbance or due to the chemical nature of particular foods. As the fellowship's cofounder, Rozanne S., describes in her history, *Beyond Our Wildest Dreams: A History of Overeaters Anonymous as Seen by a Cofounder,* a strong faction of members saw compulsive overeating as a psychosocial problem; they believed that the central aim of the twelve-step program was to redress the emotional problems that fueled the need to overeat.

Another group within OA, many of whom were recovered alcoholics from AA, viewed the root of compulsive overeating as a physical craving for food. They maintained that a chemical dependency could occur with food, just as it did with alcohol or other drugs, and that the same methods used to treat alcohol and drug addictions would be the most effective for treating food addictions.

What little research exists measuring OA's efficacy indicates that the latter approach works best. One study of 162 OA members found that those with the most success at taming their overeating were following an abstinence-based food plan.[5] These members were also more likely to report that they had never or rarely relapsed. Among a smaller sample of thirty stable OA members (defined as those with five to twenty years of recovery and weight loss), 91 percent reported abstaining from sugar, 67 percent weighed and measured their food, and 74 percent had eliminated flour, wheat, or all grains.

So, those who supported the chemical dependency theory of food addiction felt that complete abstinence from addictive foods should be the first priority of any treatment plan. Overeaters Anonymous, they declared, would create what the twelve-step literature called the "psychic change" that was necessary to ensure *long-term* recovery, but abstinence got the recovery process started in the first place. Those who claimed to be in recovery without needing to abstain from their trigger food, the chemical dependency group argued, were in denial about the true nature of their disease. Meanwhile, the psychosocial-emotional group contended that too much focus on physical abstinence turned the OA program into a mere diet.

Looking at these historical controversies among the mutual-support fellowships and professionals, we can now see that they were behaving similarly to the three blind men attempting to describe an elephant. One man feels the trunk and believes the elephant is snake-like, another feels the leg and imagines the elephant to be as big as a tree. After running into the sleeping elephant's large body, the third claims the creature is actually some type of large rock. Each bases his conclusion on only part of the whole.

How does this analogy work? Those OA members who were helped by therapists to resolve underlying trauma tended to see everyone as having similar emotional problems. After all, a survey of OA members showed that over 80 percent of the members report prior psychological, emotional, or sexual abuse, or some combination of the three. Those who found the therapeutic approach unsuccessful were considered to have not yet resolved the core issues that led them to eat compulsively.

Those who found recovery by completely eliminating sugar or wheat or other trigger foods alternatively assumed that the members who were claiming to be "in recovery" were actually expressing the denial so typical of addicts. They did not believe that it was possible to treat overeating with an "inside-out" approach of addressing internal issues first before becoming abstinent. Instead, they argued, an "outside-in" approach was necessary: people had to become abstinent first, and then they could address the internal issues that needed to be dealt with in order to maintain food sobriety. We now know that the problem with compulsive overeating and obesity is more complex than these debates suggest. *Obesity, eating disorders,* and *chemical dependency on food* are three distinct and very different diseases — and involve different behaviours around food. We can categorize the corresponding behaviours of these conditions as problems that occur within the *normal eating, emotional eating,* and *food addiction* spectrums.

Obesity is entirely a physical problem: a result of eating too many calories while expending too few. There are any number of factors that can serve as causes for the condition, factors that might upset the body's natural balance, such as hormonal or genetic irregularities. A person with a hypoactive thyroid will have a low metabolism and will not burn off calories as quickly as someone with a normal thyroid. Weight gain is the consequence. As we have seen in previous chapters, the hunger/satiety hormones of insulin and leptin can be misaligned, causing a person to feel hungry and eat more than their body's caloric need requires. Dr. Robert Lustig, in his excellent book *Fat Chance: Beating the Odds against Sugar, Processed Food, Obesity and Disease,* spells out a complex web of factors both internal and external (advertising, the careful placement of trigger foods in grocery stores, etc.) that can work to sabotage our attempts to lose weight. If these factors can be identified, it is possible to map out strategies to mitigate them and thus manage obesity successfully.

People we designate as "normal eaters" are found in the obese category. Normal eaters simply eat too much, doing so because of internal factors, such as hormones, or external influences, such as triggers (Lustig talks about our current "obeseogenic" eating environment, which strains willpower). Normal eaters represent a large proportion of the obese. They can regulate their obesity by learning how to change their circumstances to foster stronger willpower: better sleep, stress management, improving social skills, and changing a toxic food environment are only a few of the modifications that can be made. Often, simply educating a person on food choices and coaching a person to make good decisions is all that is required to successfully treat their obesity.

Certainly, people suffering from eating disorders and food addiction can also be obese, but their *primary* condition is not obesity. In their case, obesity is just another symptom of their emotional disturbance or their food addiction. The underlying emotional trauma that drives the bulimic to stuff himself needs to be addressed before the physical aspects of obesity can be treated; likewise, the sugar that is propelling the addictive overeater needs to be removed before tackling any weight issues. Once these primary conditions are addressed, there is a greater likelihood of success.

Though there are some similarities, eating disorders such as anorexia, bulimia, and binge eating disorder are, in essence, completely different from the chronic disease of obesity. Eating disorders are a result of psychological conditions, rather than strictly physical ones. The eating patterns that arise from these conditions are typically dictated by emotional needs, and can be regulated, and even resolved, if the underlying emotional disturbances are dealt with. We can call those affected by these disorders *emotional eaters*.

Chemical dependency on food, what we commonly refer to as *food addiction*, is a brain disorder caused by the interaction of trigger foods on the brains of humans predisposed to addiction. To treat food addicts, it is necessary to detoxify their brains, removing from their diets the trigger food that they crave. This is followed by education about the disease, introduction to resources for ongoing abstinence, and, only if indicated, professional treatment. No amount of physical treatment by way of drugs, hormonal manipulation, surgery, or emotional work will redress food addiction unless the chemical need for the drug is removed first.

It is, of course, possible that a person can be suffering from two, or all three, of these conditions. While there are many emotional eaters and food addicts who are normal weight, there are probably more who are also obese. The complex presentations of each of these conditions have contributed to the confusion and misdiagnoses surrounding food addiction. Clearly, one size does not fit all when it comes to obesity or disordered eating or food addiction.

The most convincing argument that obesity, emotional eating, and food addiction are separate diseases comes from a "proof is in the pudding" approach. If the treatment for a specific disease works, the diagnosis is appropriate. We are still unclear about the cause of many mental disorders, but we pragmatically make assumptions about the neurochemistry of mental illness based on the success of our treatments. For instance, we know that serotonin plays a major role in mood, because medications that alter serotonin can relieve depression. The successful management of each of these three maladies tells us a great deal about their similarities and their distinctions.

Normal Eaters

We can assume that if a person treated for obesity with a prescription for diet modification and exercise successfully loses weight and maintains that loss for years, that person is likely a normal eater. Enticing success stories in the popular media highlight this phenomenon. The "big losers," such as former Arkansas governor Mike Huckabee, singers Marie Osmond and Jennifer Hudson, actress and television host Ricki Lake, fast-food pitchman Jared Fogle ("The Subway Guy"), and Sarah Ferguson — better known as Fergie, the Duchess of York and Weight Watchers spokesperson — are some notable examples. Another celebrity is Oprah Winfrey, who actually purchased a 10-percent stake in Weight Watchers in 2015.

Sarah Ferguson, for example, who weighed two hundred pounds in 1990, lost fifty pounds while following the Weight Watchers program. She has blamed her weight problems on eating to manage painful emotions. "My parents divorced when I was twelve years old," she said, "and to cope I started eating my favourite comfort foods. I'd gain weight, take great pains to lose it, only to regain it." Even today, when she feels overtired or stressed, her mind still turns to food, looking for the comfort it gives. But Weight Watchers, she said, has taught her to recognize the warning signs and to deal with the emotions head on. "There are good days and bad days. Food is always going to be an issue for me. But I've learned to be patient and honest with myself. And if I fall off my diet, I know how to get back on track without beating myself up."[6] Janet, who we met in Chapter 2, fits into this category. When she was motivated to follow her Weight Watchers diet, she lost weight for as long as she followed her program. A fair chunk of the population fits into this category as well. According to an in-depth survey taken in 2013 by over nine thousand subscribers to *Consumer Reports* magazine, 10 to 30 percent of those who attended commercial weight loss programs lost substantial weight and kept it off for over a year.[7] A systemic review of multiple commercial diet programs (Weight Watchers, Jenny Craig, Nutrisystem, OPTIFAST, Atkins) in 2015 reported similar findings that members had notable weight loss at the one-year mark.[8]

I am also reminded of my friend Maureen, who joined me at my local Indian restaurant a few weeks ago. She is a petite, slim woman, and as she chose the lamb curry from the buffet, she told me that ten years ago she had been quite overweight. This surprised me. She tore off a piece of naan as she told me what inspired her to change her poor diet. She described how she got tired of having sore knees from marching up and down the stairs and an aching back whenever she sat for too long. She also hated feeling tired all the time. Fed up and determined to make a dietary change, she went to a nutritionist from whom she learned which food choices to limit and how to cut back on her food portions. She lost over eighty pounds *and kept it off*. I tried to imagine what eighty extra pounds would look like on her slight build. Today she still eats her favourite treats, but she controls her portions. I noticed that she only went back to the buffet one time after the initial serving, and her plate sizes were not overflowing. She shook her head when I asked her if she weighed herself on a regular basis. She knew there was a problem when her clothes began to feel too snug. If that happened, she simply cut back on the breads and pastas. Most of the time, she consciously eats a healthy diet of greens and chicken breast or fish. From her vantage point, anyone who continues to eat despite ill health isn't trying hard enough, or maybe just isn't scared enough of the consequences. Given her success, there is no reason to assume that she has an eating disorder or a food addiction. She is content with her food choices and her current weight. When normal eaters, such as Maureen or Janet, struggle with their weight or eating behaviours, they usually say that it is a matter of poor willpower because, when motivated, they just put down the fork and push away from the table. Normal eaters may like junk food, but they are usually able to weigh their priorities. The negative consequences of poor dietary choices eventually outweigh the pleasures of tasty foods. Most family physicians, and programs like Jenny Craig or Weight Watchers, base their advice to those trying to lose weight on the belief that we are all normal eaters. They encourage willpower and subtly imply that those who continue to eat are at fault.

Emotional Eaters

Most people admit to overeating sometimes in order to comfort and soothe difficult emotions. Food does provide comfort. Infants given sugar get the same analgesic effect as if they were given Aspirin. It is only when this normal coping mechanism becomes overused to the point of physical distress — obesity, diabetes, and hypertension — that normal eaters seek out help. In contrast, emotional eaters are distinctly different. They eat regardless of the pleasure of food. They are primarily eating to self-medicate, to numb unwanted feelings, usually those of anxiety, anger, or depression. The pleasure of the treat, such as the thrill of the first bite of chocolate or the burst of a citrus candy, is secondary to the need to soothe and comfort emotional unrest. The emotional eater will choose junk foods over healthy foods, not because these items taste good, but for the feeling of comfort they bring. Junk foods are designed to give feelings of warmth and safety, to dull thinking, and to settle butterflies in the stomach. To sum up: the emotional eater's primary underlying problem is not physical but mental and emotional. *It's not what you are eating but, rather, what is eating you.*

By the time emotional eaters seek medical attention, their need for food has usually become quite pathological. Since their eating behaviour has become a primary mechanism to cope with psychic distress, their symptoms have advanced to the degree that they are usually diagnosed with an eating disorder such as bulimia or binge eating disorder.

I met Karen when she was in her early twenties and had just finished the Toronto Eating Disorder program. She had spent the previous four years trying, without success, to control her binges on her own. During that first consultation with me, she described in graphic detail what she would eat: a loaf of bread, a bag of doughnuts, boxes of cookies, and chocolates. Then she would get on her exercise bike and pedal for hours, or she would purge, vomiting the food immediately after eating it: purge and then fill up again as the binge continued. By the time she came to the eating disorder clinic, she was bingeing and purging about eight times a day and was continuously obsessed by thoughts of food. Despite her compensatory measures of exercise or purging, she gradually gained weight. The unstoppable weight gain would frighten her into another binge of eating, with the inevitable purge to follow.

At the clinic, her therapist believed Karen's family dynamics were likely the root cause of her problems and encouraged her to examine them. Even as a child, she had had a tendency to put on weight, and she couldn't remember when her mother hadn't urged her to stay slim. Karen was even invited to join her mother whenever she dieted. Together, they would compare daily calorie counts and weekly weight markers. Karen admitted that, although she felt pressured to participate in her mother's diets, she was also proud of how close they became during these ventures.

Occasionally, her mother would switch tactics and entice her to eat baked goods, on holidays or whenever she felt like cooking "something special." Karen ate the food in an attempt to please her mother, but she felt confused when her mother would admonish her for gaining weight. "What did she expect?" said Karen, shrugging helplessly as she told me about it. She did not know what to do: gain the weight, or deal with the guilt and hostility that her mother exuded if she tried to refuse.

"Why did she do this?" asked Karen. "Was she trying to set me up?" Gradually, with the help of one-on-one counselling and group therapy, she learned how to recognize her anger and connect this to her binges. She also learned how to stand up to her mother, and found that the eating disorder resolved itself.

The educational sessions at the day program taught Karen that 20 percent of people who attend an eating disorder clinic eventually die of their disease. Determined not to become a statistic, she readily adopted the tools to control her eating that her therapist provided. She acquired cognitive therapy techniques that helped her monitor her bingeing thoughts and counteract her purging impulses. She learned how to eat mindfully, slowly, and thoughtfully, rather than rapidly shoveling food down her throat. Having already discovered that eating rapidly could turn a normal dinner into a voracious binge, she learned to eat a wide variety of foods, but in moderation.

Karen was also taught that eliminating specific foods, such as desserts or high fat treats, would lead to feelings of deprivation. Knowing that this could spark another relapse, she was too serious about her recovery to risk it. She saw that once her troubled family dynamics had been addressed, she was able to modify her eating behaviours so that she could stop being afraid of food and eating.

The last time I saw Karen a few years ago, her bulimia was still in remission. She continued to live with daily urges to overindulge or purge, especially when faced with an inviting buffet table or when she was tempted to share a tantalizing dessert, but there had been no significant relapses. It was a constant battle, she admitted, but most of the time she was winning. The cravings no longer seemed to daunt her.

Just as remarkable was her acceptance of being slightly "chunky." She was adamant that she would rather maintain her current weight than risk starting another cycle of binges and purges. She had been keeping tabs on the other women in her group and knew that eight of the ten had relapsed. One of the women had even died. Karen counted herself as one of the few who had truly recovered from this disorder.

Eating Disorders

Karen's experience is typical of the individual properly diagnosed with an eating disorder. Her emotional eating was treated as a symptom of a deep-seated emotional disturbance. People suffering from eating disorders typically have a childhood history of sexual abuse, a neglectful environment or, as in Karen's case, a parental environment with few clear boundaries enforced. The treatment must include a therapeutic program that deals with the underlying emotional needs that are driving the eating disorder. Often medication is included to support this goal.

Classes in the eating disorder program also teach techniques to deal with the symptoms of the disorder itself. These range from cognitive therapy techniques and mindfulness eating practices, to faith-based guidance and support groups. The intention is to disempower the individual's attitude about food from that of comfort and fear, to one of the safe, nutritional substance it actually is. Patients are taught to feel safe with all foods, rather than impose on food more emotional significance than it actually possesses.

That's why there is a deliberate attempt to include *all* foods in the treatment plan. Complete abstinence from binge foods is contraindicated. Eating disorder therapists believe that abstinence will make patients feel deprived, leading to a relapse of the disordered eating. No food should be seen as "good," "bad," or "dangerous." Healthy foods, junk foods, desserts, snacks — all are integrated into the plan so as not to encourage a pathological focus on food. Control of the eating behaviour is sought through moderation, rather than abstinence.

Portion control is taught, but this too is monitored carefully. Weighing and documenting the caloric content of foods is interpreted as an extreme measure that can trigger a diet mentality and a return to the obsession with food. It can even encourage a new eating disorder; it is not uncommon for a bulimic to acquire anorexic tendencies or an anorexic to have bulimic episodes. It can foster the eating disorder of orthorexia, which occurs when a person becomes obsessed with eating healthy foods to the point that their wellbeing is threatened. The sufferer may end up cutting all sugar, carbs, fat, meat, dairy to the point where nourishment and health are compromised.

Studies have shown that this approach works for over 60 percent of bulimics who seek treatment in this type of setting. We can find first-person accounts of success from celebrities such as actress Portia de Rossi, actress and former gymnast Cathy Rigby, and Princess Diana.[9]

For those who have not succeeded or who repeatedly relapse, the disorder itself is blamed. It is widely known that there is a high recidivism rate for eating disorders. This is especially true for the anorexic.[10] Clinicians estimate that one-third will not recover from their eating disorder, and another third, like Karen, will retain sub-threshold symptoms. Only one-third are expected to fully recover.[11]

But how do we determine success? Why do relapses occur? Is it that the person suffering from the disorder is not constantly working at managing the disorder? But what if the emotional pathology is just too deeply rooted to make a dent in the overlying symptoms of the eating disorder? Or, what if there is something else operating alongside — or even *instead of* — deep emotional distress? I believe that, one day, a missing piece of the puzzle will be found that will explain the all-too-common relapses that occur with normal eaters and emotional eaters. Perhaps it will be discovered that there is an aspect of food addiction at play.

The next chapter will provide you with an example of a food addict. You will see that even though Lawrence is morbidly obese and has deeply-rooted emotional issues, it's still the addiction dynamic that is directing his food intake — Lawrence is a food addict.

CHAPTER SEVEN

LAWRENCE:
THE TRAGIC STORY OF A FOOD ADDICT

On the sidewalk in front of Lawrence's home, I look up at an art gallery's floor-to-ceiling windows filled with eye-catching contemporary pottery and unusual artifacts. A yuppie-style gallery on the first floor of a sooty, factory-like building? Is this a building that is in the process of gentrification, soon to be full of loft units?

Walking through a doorway into the building itself, I find a huge, dark, dirty warehouse, with junk stacked high to the ceilings. There are no elevators, so I begin walking up four flights of wide cement stairs, manoeuvring past old wooden chairs and engine parts. Boxes are piled atop boxes, with blankets, books, and old bike parts spilling out. It is a picker's paradise.

As I turn the corner on the third floor, leading to the top floor and the home of my new patient, the stairwell becomes darker and narrower, with even greater piles of stuff. It is as if I am entering the centre of a web that may soon enclose its occupant.

I am about to meet Lawrence for the first time.

Friends of his had pleaded with me to come and assess him. He had become a shut-in junkie, they said, a man so obese that he was literally unable to walk, to move from his bed, let alone out of his bedroom. He sold narcotics to feed his own addiction, but he had run out of customers and was too obese to get out to hustle for new ones. Without customers, he could not afford his own habit. The irony was that he was also too obese to withdraw from his drugs: the vomiting, the diarrhea, the stress of withdrawal on his heart could kill him. I was asked to treat an addict hooked on heroin. I was about to meet a full-blown food addict.

His friends Linda and Mitch, who were both patients of mine, had also told me that his depression was just as disabling as his physical condition. Lawrence could not bear to have people see him in his present state. It mortified him to think about running into people he knew years ago, afraid of their shock at seeing what he had become. Despite his ill health, replete with episodes of chest pain and near-death overdoses, he had not left his house to get medical care or even the drugs he needed. He was just too embarrassed. But he needed a doctor to prescribe methadone to substitute for his heroin and to treat all the other ailments he had ignored over the fifteen years that he had been a recluse.

When I enter his room at the top of the last flight of stairs, it is like entering a cavern. Boxes are piled up to the vaulted ceiling, encircling a central area. Beyond a threadbare but elaborate oriental carpet stands a king-size bed.

On top of the bed sits Lawrence.

Lawrence, who turns out to be in his early fifties, is the biggest man I've ever seen. He is propped up like a Buddha, with an Aztec-style smock draped over him from shoulders to feet. Almost six hundred pounds, he fills half of the bed. A large iron ring hangs from the ceiling, which he uses to hoist himself up when he sees me. Oddly enough, my first impression is not of his enormous body, but of his larger-than-life personality. A broad smile crosses his face and he raises a massive arm to greet me.

"Doctor," he says, beaming. "How good of you to come! So glad you came. Thank you, thank you."

A man with charm, I think. I can see how Lawrence had at one time been a player, a trader and seller in the antique world, as his friends said.

Lawrence motions to a rake-thin man hovering nearby, almost hidden in the shadows. "This is Frank, a friend who helps me out."

He points toward the kitchen, a makeshift affair that has no door. (Really, it's just a corner of the loft with a fridge, stove, and table covered in kitchen items.)

"Get her something to drink. Do we have any tea?"

I pull a stethoscope from my medical bag. I wonder about this man who fetches the tea with a tentative nod toward me and then shrinks back into a dark corner of the room. Turning to Lawrence, I prepare to ask him my list of questions about his drug addiction. After that, I intend to do a thorough physical. How will I test his blood pressure on those huge arms, though? My large cuff won't encircle his biceps.

Lawrence wants to talk. I can tell by his quick and easy way with words that he is an extrovert by nature, eager to engage with others. Years ago, he tells me, he was a world traveller, making a good life for himself by collecting unusual items that he would clean, repair, and sell to the Queen Street shops in the funky west end of Toronto. Some of his better finds were included in the gallery downstairs. He starts to tell me about his life in New York, where he lived before he came to Toronto.

I realize that more than twenty minutes have passed and I still haven't acquired the information that I need. When I ask him a question about his drug use, he launches into another digression related to his past life, this time when he was an art collector living the high life on cocaine. Listening, I wonder if he is now a squatter who refuses to move from the top floor of what had once been his studio. Linda told me that the owner of the building, which is a choice piece of real estate, sitting one block away from the Art Gallery of Ontario, has wanted to sell the warehouse for some time, but he hasn't the heart to tell Lawrence to go. Where would he possibly go?

I can see that Lawrence is very proud of the esoterica he has collected over the years. Amidst the old broken engines, boxes, and textiles lie small woven Peruvian blankets, multi-coloured and braided Columbian hats, and straw dolls. He insists that his collection of South American dolls alone, if repaired, is worth a great deal of money. I look around and spot the dolls huddled in rows in an open wooden cabinet. Dwarfing these are piles upon piles of *National Geographic* magazines, out-of-print rare books, comic books, and unusual drug paraphernalia, everything in large piles scattered here and there on the floor.

Lawrence tells me that he lived in New York in the mid-1980s and made a thriving business for himself in the art community there. He proudly says he had a gallery of his own at one point and even a following of people who were captivated by his lifestyle. Those were the days when he used cocaine to fuel his busy lifestyle and, knowing that he had a tendency to gain weight, to control his weight. Then he moved to Toronto. No longer in the hub of the art world, he lost his network of contacts for his business. Eventually, he started dealing drugs instead. It was quick and easy money. Over time, he developed a different social network, one that was more drug- than art-related.

Unlike the stereotype of the junkie, Lawrence gained weight on heroin. Instead of running around wheeling and dealing, burning off excess calories with cocaine, he drifted through large portions of his day alone in a stupor. His major source of income soon became selling drugs from his home. Lawrence would buy a large quantity of drugs from a dealer, divide it into small quantities to sell, and keep a portion for his own use. People would come over at all times of the day and night, stomping up the stairs under the direction of Frank, and meet Lawrence here at his bedside. He sold them their drugs and often they would spend the evening with him, keeping him company, sharing their drugs. Together, they nattered and nodded off into blissful reveries in this cool loft filled with so many curiosities. At times, it seemed an enchanted life.

But inactivity was bad for Lawrence. To his mortification, his weight just kept increasing. Soon he began avoiding people, reluctant to leave the house because he was fearful of their disdain. When his drug customers stopped coming around so often, Lawrence became increasingly isolated. Within ten years of moving to Toronto, he had become a shut-in. By the time that I met him, he had not been out of his home in seven years. With the exception of Frank, Linda, and Mitch, he had not seen anyone for two weeks. And in that seven years he had gained more than three hundred pounds.

His spindly friend Frank turned out to be an alcoholic, with an odd manner that was both obsequious and fearful. I couldn't tell if he was an old friend or a freeloader who happened to find shelter from living on the street by acting as Lawrence's gopher. Lawrence was ambivalent toward him; sometimes he responded warmly to the thin man's presence, while at other times he seemed almost contemptuous. Over the time that I met with Lawrence, I learned that Frank bought Lawrence's groceries and prepared the food that they ate together. The odd time drug addicts came to buy from Lawrence, he would escort them up the stairs. Since it took almost superhuman effort for Lawrence to get up — he was terrified he would fall and be unable to get up (and his slight friend would be of little help) — the thin man would even fetch his toilet pail.

Lawrence had not seen a doctor in seven years. He had no idea if his blood pressure was high or if he was a diabetic, and, moreover, he did not want to know. He admitted that he had had episodes of chest pain in the past that concerned him, but he had refused to call an ambulance. Once, years ago, an emergency response team had been called. Lawrence had felt humiliated when they cursed and muttered that the narrow stairwells were a hazard. They warned him that they would not come back until the mounds of debris were cleared. Lawrence had no idea how he would accomplish that task. Frank took stabs at doing this from time to time, and, when he did, he would often be out of sight amidst the mountains of boxes for hours.

Eventually, this state of affairs became untenable. Lawrence could no longer afford his drug addiction as fewer customers came by, and the means of supporting his habit shrank. OxyContin and crack had replaced heroin as the drugs of choice on the streets, neither of which he had access to. (To obtain them required being out on the streets, hustling and visiting multiple doctors to get the supply he needed for his opiate dependence.) Now, he worried about surviving a heroin withdrawal. How would he cope with violent diarrhea and vomiting? Going to a detox centre was out of the question.

That's why Lawrence wanted to get methadone, to avoid the shock of quitting cold turkey. His last reliable customers, my patients Linda and Mitch, had guiltily told him one day that they had decided to get off drugs and would take methadone instead. They knew that Lawrence would lose the last crumbs of drug income to buy his own drugs if they left. That's when they told him they would ask me if I could help him the way I had helped them.

After some deliberation on my part, and lots of charm on his, I agreed to take him on as a patient. Because he could not come to my office, I came to his home once a week to prescribe him methadone. While he was stabilizing on methadone, I was expected to monitor him regularly to ensure that he was getting the correct prescription. I had to check his vitals and test his urine at least weekly.

Over the course of the next six months, I tried to help Lawrence with his heroin addiction as well as his other medical needs. I always intended to stay only twenty minutes, but it was difficult to get the information I needed because of Lawrence's obsessive need to talk. He was isolated, and I was sometimes the only person he saw in a day. We discussed his past, his frustrations, and his hopes for the future. We discussed his drug use and what he might do if he could shake his addiction. Our sessions ended up lasting more than an hour each week.

Getting the methadone to Lawrence was not an easy task, as he had no way of getting to the pharmacy on a daily basis. For a while, the pharmacist gallantly came by every day to deliver the medication, but this was not a permanent solution. It was important that Lawrence get clean from his drug use, but his urine samples continued to show positive for opiates and cocaine. Lawrence was clearly still using and did not show any signs of letting up.

His housemate must have been bringing drugs to Lawrence. How else was he getting them? I wasn't even sure how Lawrence could afford to keep using without Linda and Mitch. Was he still dealing? When I confronted Lawrence about his ongoing use, he blamed Frank. "He wants me to keep using so I'll stay dependent on him," he whispered. Then he smiled disarmingly. "Anyway, I can't stop," he said. "What have I got? TV and drugs. What else am I supposed to do?"

I could see what he meant.

I urged Lawrence to lose weight. It seemed like a monumental task, but I naively believed if he recovered his mobility, his options to find other sources of pleasure besides TV and drugs would expand. If he could get out, meet with old friends, I thought, he might find reasons to stay sober. I proposed a diet and promised to coach him. He listened to my proposed food plan, nodding, excited to try out the new regimen. He would try anything I suggested, and together we came up with what I thought was a realistic food plan that would enable him to lose weight.

Yet, each time I visited, it was obvious to me that he had neither stopped using drugs nor curbed his eating.

"What about the plan?" I asked impatiently. The weeks were dragging on.

He shrugged. He was trying, he said, sighing and looking down at his massive body.

I tried hypnosis, but that proved no more successful at stopping Lawrence's drug use or his eating. One thing he loved, though, was the long script that I read to him each time I came. He said the affirmations made him feel free of the shame and self-loathing that shrouded his days. By way of showing his gratitude, he insisted that I pick out a few of his prized possessions. Once, I left with an embroidered hat and a carved walking stick. As I felt the unusual texture of the bark on the stick and told him how impressed I was, he beamed.

After three months, his drug use eventually slowed down. But it seemed that his eating got worse. Lawrence explained that he just got too depressed if he didn't have *something* to occupy his long days and even longer evenings. I suggested that we try antidepressants, but he protested that he did not want "stuff to mess up my mind." While that may sound curious for a man who abused opiates and cocaine, it is typical of addicts in Lawrence's age group. (Today, young addicts are only too eager to get meds.)

I asked Linda and Mitch, who still came to keep him company, not to bring him treats. ("But he keeps asking us, how can we say no?" they groaned.) I also asked Frank — when I could find him, since he always slunk away when I came — not to enable Lawrence by buying items that I'd put on our forbidden food list. The thin man shrugged shamefacedly when I suggested this, but I knew he still brought Lawrence forbidden food. By now, my consultations with Lawrence had become fixed hour-long sessions as I tried to build his self-esteem and identify the obstacles that were holding back his therapeutic progress.

Over time, our discussions about dieting became shorter and less frequent as I grew increasingly frustrated. I was also aware that I was not helpful anymore: rather than encouraging Lawrence toward a brighter future, I found myself bullying or scolding him. He said he wanted to change his eating patterns and lose weight, but did he really want to? I was not convinced.

Sadly, Lawrence died of a heart attack nine months after we began our weekly visits. I received the call from Linda, who was one of the last people to keep in contact with Lawrence. She was still coming by to bring him food, since she did not trust Frank. As I put the phone down, I stared absently at the walls of my office.

I had mixed feelings. In a way, I felt relieved that an untenable situation had resolved itself. Lawrence's pharmacist had told me earlier that week that he had to stop coming to Lawrence's house to dispense the methadone. The official requirements of the methadone program are that if a person is still using drugs, as Lawrence still was, he had to get his methadone dispensed *daily* by a pharmacist. Lawrence was on the verge of having to deal with an abrupt cessation of methadone, and that withdrawal is worse than heroin withdrawal.

I also felt a great deal of sadness. Lawrence was an intriguing man. The work of treating addictions is often intense, and the doctor-patient relationship can be strong. In the course of treating Lawrence I had come to know him well. I knew I would miss him terribly. I looked up and saw the row of *National Geographic* DVDs — a set that comprised every issue since the magazine launched decades ago. I hadn't wanted them, but I knew that Lawrence needed to give me something from his stash of collectables that he deemed precious.

Lawrence was only fifty-three years old when he died. He had managed to reduce his drug use from several times a day to a few times a week. Given the circumstances, that was a remarkable badge of success. Maybe he even cut down on his food consumption, but how could I really know? I could not determine if he had lost any weight, as I had never been able to weigh him. But I believed that my interventions had made a difference.

I heard from his friends that removing the body from the building fulfilled Lawrence's worst nightmare: the paramedics had to break down the doorframe to get his body out of the loft. Linda also told me that Frank had disappeared, taking some of the most valuable items in the apartment with him.

At Lawrence's visitation, I saw some of the friends he'd known just before he became reclusive. Most of them looked as if they had been his drug customers, the ones who would stay at his place to get high together. They were huddled in groups of three and four, talking amongst themselves. I wondered if I should identify myself as his doctor in the last year of his life. Would they care? Occasionally, we would individually go up to the coffin and look at Lawrence's large body, a rosary held in his folded hands. Then we would retreat back to our couches and watch each other or newcomers who entered the room. I wondered if Frank would show up.

Linda and Mitch sat with me, reluctant to converse with the others. They had stopped using drugs and did not want to associate with anyone else in the room. They spoke again about the tragedy of Lawrence's life: how he had been a rising star at one time, only to turn to heroin and lose his edge in the art world. The weight he had gained during his final years seemed a cruel finish to the life of such a charismatic and generous man. Then the topic of conversation turned to more practical matters. Who would go through the mountains of junk before the landlord carted it all away to a dumpster? How soon could they get into the loft before Frank stole even more of the valuables hidden amidst the junk? They wondered whether they could even store whatever they did find. Lawrence had left behind just too much stuff.

Are all food addicts destined to end up like Lawrence? Does it need to get *this* bad? I use Lawrence's story because his life illustrates a particularly stark, extreme version of the final stage of food addiction, where we imagine most food addicts will end up if they do not seek treatment. You will see in the next chapters more versions of this same terrible trajectory. Though extreme, Lawrence's story is not unusual.

Is it possible to diagnose food addicts earlier in their affliction, before so much damage is done? I believe so, but first the disease must be identified. This is not always easy to do, since its appearance can differ depending on how advanced the illness is. As we have already seen, the different expressions of obesity and eating behaviours can create confusion even for the most astute clinicians.

Early diagnosis provides a window of opportunity. With the right intervention, it's possible to slow down the progression of the illness in early-stage food addicts. Obesity, cross addictions, diabetes, and depression can be averted if food addicts simply "get off the bus" of their addiction sooner rather than later, if they can stop eating the foods that propel their addiction and drive the circumstances of their lives further into the ground.

To discover how a diagnosis of food addiction can be made, it's helpful to see how the addiction can manifest itself over the course of a lifetime. What are the telltale danger signs? That will be the focus of the next chapter.

CHAPTER EIGHT

STAGES OF FOOD ADDICTION

The best way to appreciate the different stages of food addiction, following the excellent work of Phil Werdell, is to see how they play out in the life of a food addict.[1] Here are two stories to show what food addiction looks like. Hopefully, they will help other food addicts recognize their own addiction. Once they are able to recognize the telltale signs that appear in each phase of the addiction, they might be willing to consider consulting an addictions counsellor before it is too late. Why not get off the bus sooner rather than later?

Stephanie's Story

Pre-Disease Phase

Until Stephanie was in her early teens, she did not have any major difficulties with food. She had no problem making the transition from breastfeeding to eating soft foods to solid foods. She ate everything she was given, showing no particular attachment to sweets. Stephanie did not seem to care if she ate dessert or not. Once, in elementary school, she ate four root beer Popsicles and got a stomach ache. She never did that again.

So, Stephanie binged once, but it was a one-time incident, and after resolving not to repeat it, she did not think anything about it again. Generally a happy girl, she liked reading and playing soccer, and did well in school. She enjoyed going to church, participated actively in the children's choir, and usually had a part in the holiday plays. She had at least two close girlfriends and they often stayed over at each other's homes.

So far, this could be the story of a normal child who, like many kids, overate to the point of stomach upset once. It could alternatively be the story of a girl with a nascent food addiction.

Early Stage

Stephanie entered puberty the summer before junior high school and developed more quickly than her peers. A boy she liked told her she was fat. Was she, Stephanie worried, as she compared herself to her friends? Not wanting to gain weight, she began reducing the portions of her meals and sometimes refused to eat deep-fried foods.

In the summer between grade eight and high school, Stephanie joined a circle of friends who liked to party. They smoked pot for the first time, started drinking beer regularly, and experimented with sex. Since all of her friends were "doing it," Stephanie considered this behaviour both natural and exciting. She worried less about her weight as her friends matured and filled out.

In her first semester of high school, Stephanie seemed quite happy and well adjusted. But things changed after spring break. Suddenly, she began calling herself "Steph," retreating from her friends, and spending more time alone in her room, brooding. Her parents wondered what had happened with her boyfriend. "Oh, nothing, really," she replied. Her parents also quizzed her about her new weight gain: What was she eating? "Nothing new," she said, shrugging.

Neither answer was true.

Stephanie, who had often been bingeing on chips and cookies, had become alarmed at how quickly she was gaining weight. However, earlier that year, she had learned a new habit from her girlfriends. Some of them had been purging their meals to control their weight and Stephanie was curious to try this as well. She liked this trick of being able to eat a lot and not get fat. Stephanie and her best friend talked about it as "their secret."

At the same time, Stephanie's grades dropped. When she stopped playing sports in her senior year, her school counsellor called her into his office to express his concern. She shrugged him off, not daring to tell him about her secret or about anything else in her life. What would he have thought if she had disclosed her binges and purges to him? Would he have assumed that this was the story of a teenager temporarily caught up in doing what her friends were doing, or would he have wondered if she was in the early stage of either an eating disorder or a food addiction? Either way, Stephanie was not at a time in her life when she was prepared to deal with her issues.

Middle Stage

Steph, as she now called herself, loved the freedom she found in college life. Her marks didn't improve — she hardly opened a book all semester — but she excelled in extracurricular recreation: drinking and using drugs regularly on the weekends. She was in a crowd where "hooking up" sexually was the norm. It was party time all the time. She went from bingeing and purging once or twice a week to doing so at least once a day, sometimes more. Yet, to her dismay, she still gained weight: thirty pounds during her first three months of college. Her secret tool was not as reliable as she had come to expect.

Just before exam week, the party ended; Steph discovered she was pregnant. In a state of shock, she cried in the counsellor's office for nearly an hour, uncertain of what to do next. She finally decided to have an abortion, but did not know how she would cope with the experience. Electing to drop out of college and go home for a few months to get "her head back on straight," she quit drinking and smoking pot, although she continued overeating.

Within a week of returning home, her bulimia spiralled out of control. She purged after every meal. At night, she would sneak into the kitchen to raid the refrigerator, promising herself "just to have some leftovers from dinner or a dish of ice cream," but found that she could not stop at that. Late one night, her mother asked her what had happened to all the crackers, cookies, milk, and ice cream.

Finally, Steph told the truth.

Distressed and concerned, her parents discussed her options with her and helped her find the best eating disorder counsellor in town. Steph was relieved to be able to unburden herself: she revealed her secrets to the therapist, who taught her new ways to deal with her feelings without using food. After several months of therapy, Steph confessed to what had been bothering her since her senior year in high school.

Steph had gone to a hotel one night that year with a young man she liked and trusted, feeling safe in his company. But after they'd stepped into the room, he locked the door behind them and turned to her with an angry face. "If you tell even one person," he hissed, "I'll kill you." He then brutally raped her.

Feeling humiliated and ashamed, Steph told no one about the incident, not even her best friend. Now, with the support of her therapist, she felt she was ready to talk. She told her family in a group session with her therapist and later accused the man, even testifying at his trial. It turned out she was not the only young woman he had molested, and, to her relief, he was convicted. Although the process had been difficult, she finally felt free of the burden of a secret trauma that had stained her past until then. Having reclaimed her past, she even stopped going by "Steph" and became Stephanie again.

This could clearly be the story of a young woman with a trauma-based eating disorder. If so, the treatment for her condition was appropriate. But was it the right thing for Stephanie? I don't think so. As you will see, Stephanie was not able to moderate her binges and purges, despite this successful therapeutic intervention. I believe she had a progressive food addiction. Had Stephanie learned about Overeaters Anonymous or one of the other food-related twelve-step programs, I think she might have halted the progression of her disease at this point.

Late Stage

The following year, Stephanie returned to college and applied herself academically. Her grades turned around, and she even made it to the Dean's List. She also tried out for soccer, winning an athletic scholarship a year later. It took her a while to return to dating, but eventually she met someone she really liked. They took it slowly and, by their junior year, they were going steady.

Stephanie was proud of herself. Studying social work felt like a good fit for her, and she was happy with the way her life seemed to be on track. But there was just one problem. About once a week, Stephanie "treated" herself to a binge. And during exam periods, she would treat herself more often, to help her get through the grind of endless study. At first, she was very careful not to purge, as she did not want to relapse into her old bulimic behaviour. But when she started to notice that her clothes were a bit too tight, she decided it would be all right again to use her "secret weapon".

By the time Stephanie was in graduate school, she was back to binge-ing and purging almost every day. She admitted it to a group of friends but assured them she was managing well otherwise. She maintained a full-time job while plugging away at her degree. She kept up her relation-ship with her boyfriend, but, she told me, she was starting to find each day quite stressful, starting to find it increasingly hard to balance all her responsibilities. Eventually, she broke up with her boyfriend and told her friends that her binges had increased to daily episodes. Her friends staged an intervention and suggested she see a therapist.

Having been through it once before, Stephanie progressed quickly in therapy. She stopped purging, identified old patterns she had developed in childhood, and created a foundation for the problems she confronted in high school and college. She worked on her body image. Gradually, Stephanie rebuilt her self-confidence, intent on healing herself physically, mentally, emotionally, and spiritually. The idea of "eat when hungry, stop when full" fit with her new practices of meditation and yoga. She liked the idea of "listening to your body" as a guide to balanced eating.

Was she successful? Three years later, when Stephanie graduated with a master's degree in social work, she should have been happy, but, privately, she was distressed that she weighed more than two hundred pounds. She could not seem to shake her overeating. It seemed that her approach of eating until she was full was not working out. Most of the time she still felt hungry, even when she knew she should be full.

Nonetheless, Stephanie excelled in her professional life. She found her job working in a program for teen parents meaningful, because she felt that she was really making a difference in people's lives. She was overjoyed when her clients became success stories. Some were able to give up drugs. Most earned their high school diploma or GED. Several went on to college and fulfilling careers. During this period, Stephanie also enjoyed two relationships with men.

The only downside was her weight. By the time she turned thirty-five, she was up to two hundred and forty pounds. She did not want to have children at that weight, knowing a pregnancy could make her gain even more weight. But what could she do? She did not want to repeat her purging behaviour, and her strategy of managing her appetite had deteriorated into a dismal failure. Listening to her body, she realized, was not working. She could never eat enough ice cream or deep-dish pizza to satisfy her cravings.

A friend of Stephanie's told her about Food Addicts in Recovery Anonymous. Her friend had joined earlier that year and lost a significant amount of weight. She urged Stephanie to attend a meeting, to try it just once. Stephanie agreed and they went together the next night. She looked at all the women sitting in a circle in the room, noting that most of them were professional, courteous, and … slim. They told stories about how heavy they had been in the past and about their eating patterns. Nodding, she identified with each one of them. She carefully listened to their stories of how they had changed their lives since coming into the group. She studied their food plans.

Although she liked the program, Stephanie found its guidelines quite strict. For example, she was required to do things that had nothing to do with eating, like going to meetings and calling fellow group members regularly. Still, she decided she was willing to follow these rules as she was not sure what else to do. Since nothing else had worked, she really had nothing to lose.

The idea that she was addicted to sugar and flour was a new concept to her, although intuitively it made sense to her. So, she agreed to eliminate these foods from her daily diet. Every day she documented and revealed her food choices and portion sizes to another member of the group and she attended meetings on a weekly basis. But her irritability and obsession with food remained. She was frustrated by how difficult it was to not cheat with the junk food that seemed to occupy her mind all day. It was not until she attended a food addiction recovery workshop that offered 24/7 supports for five days that she was able to abstain for five whole days and get past the initial withdrawal symptoms. To her relief, her cravings for ice cream and pizza gradually lessened. She had never made it that long before, so the lack of cravings was a new experience for her.

Stephanie, who has stuck with her twelve-step program and lost more than one hundred pounds, now accepts that she is a food addict. With her obsessive cravings under control, she feels like her old self again. The program has worked like nothing else before.

Final Stage

Had Stephanie not found and accepted support for her food addiction, her disease would have progressed even further. She would have experienced secondary complications from her obesity. Already pre-diabetic, her blood pressure and cholesterol were on the high end of normal, so she was already at risk for heart disease or a stroke. If she had gained more weight, I expect she would eventually have had joint and back problems. Exercise would have become impossible to do. If she had considered bariatric surgery, there would have been a 30-percent chance she wouldn't have lost any weight at all, or would have regained it within a year. Instead, Stephanie continues to live an addiction-free life, abstaining from sugar and flour, and maintaining a weight she is very happy with.

Walter's Story

Pre-Disease Phase

Walter skipped the pre-disease stage. If there is such a thing as a fetus becoming addicted to food in the womb, Walter is a likely candidate. This isn't wild speculation: there are genetic markers for both addiction and obesity, indicating that some people may be genetically predisposed to both conditions. Walter's father was an active alcoholic and his mother had, at one time, been in treatment for drug addiction, so addiction was part of Walter's family history.

Walter showed signs suggesting the early stages of food addiction from the time he was born. The first indication of this was his whimper each time his mother tried to pull him away from her breast, after she determined he had more than a full feeding. His first words were *uuuu* sounds, which his parents quickly figured out meant "sugar."

Early Stage

As an infant, Walter was a non-stop eater. Like many women of her generation — a boomer who came of age in the early seventies — his mother naively believed that hunger was always a sign of health, so she fed him every chance she could. Walter was a fat baby, which his family believed indicated that he was going to grow up to be a "real man." They thought it was cute when they would see him sneaking candies from the bowl in his grandmother's living room. When Walter's doctor disagreed, suggesting the family give the boy smaller meals, his parents shrugged, telling friends, "He really just likes to eat."

Relatives also contributed to the problem. They bought Walter a Chicago Bears jersey for his first birthday, along with a box of Baby Ruth candy bars. As a two-year-old, Walter starred in a home movie as the "future football player." Once, his uncles teased him and debated whether he would turn out to be more like Walter Payton II or William "The Refrigerator" Perry, both enormous NFL football players.

Occasionally, a family member would try to curb Walter's food intake. However, whenever a giggling Walter started grabbing food from the refrigerator and his father took it away, Walter would have an all-out tantrum.

Middle Stage

By kindergarten, Walter was fifty pounds overweight and his doctor had classified him as obese. The doctor told the skeptical family that Walter was not alone in receiving this diagnosis. The rates of childhood obesity have skyrocketed in the last thirty years. Statistics indicate that one quarter of all U.S. children are overweight. The Canada Health Survey shows similarly distressing trends of childhood obesity. In 1978, only 3 percent of children between the ages of two and seventeen were obese, but by 2004 that number had skyrocketed to 12 percent, meaning that a distressingly large number of children were at high risk for diabetes and early death in their thirties and forties due to stroke or heart disease.

These statistics on childhood obesity match the trends in increased sugar consumption. In 1999, the Center for Science in the Public Interest (CSPI) noted that sugar consumption in the United States had increased 28 percent since 1983. This rise is largely attributed to sodas and sugar-sweetened fruit drinks. Our children are especially vulnerable to these alarming dietary shifts. Where the average sugar consumption of an adult is now twenty-two teaspoons a day, it is thirty-four teaspoons a day for adolescents.[2]

Walter's doctor knew that young Walter was heading toward a life of chronic illness if things did not change, and he urged the family to alter Walter's diet. He warned the parents about the potential dangers of obesity: childhood Type 2 diabetes, high cholesterol, and high blood pressure. Sadly, these are indices doctors would rarely have considered in young people years ago. Did his doctor also warn the family about the possibility that Walter might be developing a binge eating disorder at this time? Perhaps, but food addiction would probably not have been on his menu of possibilities.

When asked what he liked best about school, young Walter answered, "Snacks." He used his allowance money to buy candies from the corner store. If he ran out, he pocketed coins from his father's dresser and lied when asked about the missing change. Although he knew that it was wrong and that it could get him into serious trouble, even at this early age his compulsion to do whatever was necessary to obtain the food he craved was so strong that he would steal to buy more treats.

His typical day would begin with a hearty breakfast loaded with sugar. He especially liked Froot Loops, a cereal that contains twelve grams of sugar per one-ounce serving, to which he added sugar on top, eating this along with buttered raisin toast spread with cinnamon sugar. He also loved full-fat chocolate milk. His brothers and sisters teased him about all the sugar he consumed, telling him he was "too sweet!" But when Walter learned that "Sweetness" was the nickname of the famous football player Walter Payton, he set his sights on growing up to play professional football. Soon his friends at school nicknamed him "Big Sweet."

Although he was bright, Walter seemed distracted in class, as though schoolwork did not interest him.

"What are you thinking about?" a classmate once asked. "Lunch," he said with a laugh.

Walter had a cheery disposition that made him popular with the other kids. Still, he would get teased about his weight and he had to hide the sting he felt. When his peers said things like "Are you going to be able to fit in that desk?" or "Be careful you don't break the seats on the bus," or "Don't put a pin in Walter's butt, it'll let all the helium out," the taunts hurt him bitterly.

During his first year in high school, Walter finally tried out for football (after having been told that he was too heavy to excel at such a sport). In the football tryouts, he was offered a choice between being an offensive or a defensive tackle, rather than the position he really wanted — quarterback — but for which he was far too big. Grudgingly, Walter accepted the position. He went home, and with tears on his face, he opened the kitchen cabinet door and found what he was looking for: a big bag of Oreos that would make him feel better.

That was Walter's pattern: he would get upset, then binge on sugary, fatty foods to feel better. Every day, after practice, he raided the kitchen. His mother found that she could not keep the cupboards stocked with enough cookies and cakes. If he couldn't find sweets, Walter ate leftovers from the previous day's meals. To no one's surprise, by the end of high school he weighed three hundred pounds.

Walter felt vindicated when he got a sport scholarship for college. (He would not have been able to get into college without a scholarship.) With people applauding his success and no longer commenting on his weight, his self-esteem improved. He did not dare tell his family that he had to obtain a doctor's note allowing him to play on the team despite his weight.

For Walter, college life was all about football, working out, and eating. His coach pulled him aside at one point and said, "There's a chance that you will star on the varsity squad if you can take off at least forty pounds." Four hours of intense daily practice helped him work off those pounds and keep him at a steady weight.

While Walter had been an average student in high school, in college he found it impossible to keep up even a passing grade. He was simply too tired to stay awake in class and exercise the necessary hours needed to maintain his weight. He hired a tutor and got transferred to a special class with other football players; he even paid other students to write his papers and take his exams. He worried constantly that he might fail.

In spite of his attempt to control his weight, he continued to eat too much of the wrong things. He would tell the server at the fast-food counter, "I'm taking orders for my teammates." He would eat half the order on the way to his dorm and then finish the rest before he fell asleep. Walter knew that this would mean he would have to work out harder the next day, but he found he could not stop himself from driving back out to the nearest fast-food outlet and buying two or three orders of food each night.

Late Stage

When Walter was not recruited to play professional football, he became dejected and gradually stopped working out. He just did not have the heart for it. What was the point? Without the intense, regular exercise, he started gaining weight again. He sank into a low-grade depression that dogged him day after day. When he tried to relieve his despondency by going to the movies, he found he could lift his mood temporarily only if he had an extra-large order of buttered popcorn, a large soda, and an assortment of candy bars. He would eat the popcorn and soda quickly in order to take advantage of offers for "free seconds" on those items. He would laugh and tell friends that the characteristics all his food had in common were that they were "large" and offered "free seconds." Nevertheless, he fretted constantly about his mounting weight gain, although the more preoccupied he became with it, the more he ate.

Like most obese people, Walter hated being so overweight. Having to be careful wherever he sat down to make sure he did not break a chair. Having to travel first class to get a larger seat and asking for a seatbelt extender was embarrassing, tedious, and expensive. It was nearly impossible for him to reach his genitals when he showered. Everywhere he went, he thought people stared at him with pity or disgust. He had stopped dating long ago. Of course, he also dreaded going to the doctor and hearing the inevitable admonition: "You have to lose weight."

Walter was only thirty-two when he had his first heart attack. It frightened him enough to stop him from eating excessively, and he lost twenty-two pounds. ("Gee, I'll have to do that again," he joked.)

But to keep off the weight, he needed to change his eating patterns, which he found impossible to do. He wondered if he should get bariatric surgery.[3] When he approached his doctor, hoping this surgery could provide a new beginning for his life, his doctor agreed, but only if Walter could demonstrate first that he could eat the small portions he would be expected to eat after the surgery for the rest of his life. The realization that even after the surgery he would be on a diet for the rest of his life left Walter feeling even more hopeless. On his way home from the doctor's office he stopped at a grocery store and, later that night, ate as much as he could.

Final Stage

Walter's story does not have a happy ending. He did eventually have the bariatric surgery, but he could not stop indulging in his triple-sized meals and his love for treats like popcorn and soda. He regained the weight quickly and, after a few years, he died obese, alone, and addicted.

Stages of Food Addiction

Addiction is like an elevator that only goes down, but you can get off at any floor. It is one of the mysteries and frustrations of those of us in the addictions treatment field that one can never predict if or when an addict will disembark.

Like any addiction, food addiction is a chronic, progressive condition. As illustrated with Stephanie and Walter, there are four identifiable stages. In the early stage of the addiction, food addicts experience some loss of control, as with Stephanie's occasional food binges. Like so many in this early stage, she appeared to be a normal, healthy eater, who indulged in only occasional excesses. But something is usually different, even at this early stage. Remember the guilt Walter felt about his early binges, including the lying and stealing that supported them?

At this early stage, both Stephanie and Walter could have stopped the progression of their disease by simply not eating the binge-triggering foods. But the guilt or shame of overeating is usually not sufficient enough at this stage to justify such radical action. The food addict, like all of us, lives in a society that encourages a mutual sharing of excessive food intake: all-you-can-eat buffets, lavish holiday meals, gatherings where rich and sugary foods are highlighted. Overindulging is held to be normal in these contexts, and identifying a binge as a binge can be difficult — the label is in the eye of the beholder. So, without such a label, early-stage food addicts can easily justify their behaviour as normal.

By the middle stage of the disease, most food addicts will have gained unwanted weight and may have resorted to periodic dieting. Both Walter and Stephanie had developed routines to control their weight; Stephanie indulged in her secretive bingeing and purging and Walter used excessive exercise. Others may choose deliberate periods of restricting food intake or purging the excess calories by vomiting or using laxatives. These behaviours are typical of emotional eaters as well as food addicts. In the early stage, it would be easy to misdiagnose either Stephanie or Walter as having an eating disorder instead of a food addiction.

Middle-stage food addicts, however, engage in other behaviours *specific* to addiction. Hoarding particular foods, especially if stores don't restock preferred items quickly enough, is one red flag. (In this case, food is being treated like a drug stash.) Sometimes, food addicts steal items from stores. Also, they frequently find themselves finishing off other people's food. They almost always lie about their food — about what they eat and especially about how much of it they eat — although they are lying to themselves as much as to others. I have seen the confused look on their faces as they quiz the nutritionist: "Why am I not losing weight? Everything I eat is healthy!" They constantly underestimate their food intake. Unless asked to keep a food diary, they forget about their daily cola and morning bagel slathered with jam; they don't remember the quick grabs of candy at the office door; they forget to count the packets of sugar and dollops of whipped cream in their lattes.

As with alcoholics at this stage, they may say that they "want to want to stop," and may believe they can control their food intake — "I just need more willpower," they will say — but they cannot follow their diet, no matter how motivated.

Late-stage food addicts finally realize they have *no* control over food, although many die before they reach this stage. They deny that their diabetes, heart attacks, or strokes are a direct result of the food they have been unable to stop eating. But a small number "get it" before the downward spiral happens. They recognize the failures of previous diets, hypnosis, psychotherapy, diet clinics, and peer support groups. While there are often many benefits from talk therapy, they have learned that controlling their eating is not one of them.

Although Stephanie learned some tremendous coping skills in talk therapy, her binge eating continued. Sorting out her issues, even the traumatic rape in high school, made little difference in the long run. Walter was so ashamed of his eating that he did not tell his doctor, dietician, or therapist the full extent of his overeating. He could not bear hearing their advice to stop eating, knowing that it was impossible for him to do so. They simply did not seem to understand his struggle.

In late-stage food addiction, there are always medical consequences. As with those suffering from obesity or an advanced eating disorder, late-stage food addicts often have high blood pressure, diabetes, heart disease, depression, anxiety, and many other physical and psychological ailments. As Walter's story illustrates, people suffering from obesity are in danger of shortening their lives by five to ten years because of these conditions.

I applaud the American Medical Association, which, in 2013, officially acknowledged obesity as a chronic illness in its own right, requiring a range of medical interventions. This has led to more research into the causes and management of obesity, as well as into its consequences. But unless the underlying substance use disorder is addressed, I am concerned that this research won't help food addicts. For many extremely obese individuals, bariatric surgery, such as lap-band or gastric bypass, and even medication, can be helpful. But if they are also suffering from an advanced stage of food addiction, they are likely to start overeating again within a year, losing the benefits of surgery or medication.

Although most bariatric clinics insist on a restricted diet of less sugar and starch for a successful outcome, clinicians admit that almost 60 percent of their patients, like Walter, eventually regain their weight by the five-year mark. These patients are not able to maintain the required diet for the long haul. (It is possible that the 40 percent who are successful with surgery and diet were not food addicts, although there is not yet any empirical evidence to support this.) For bariatric surgery to be successful for a food addict, the post-treatment counselling needs to address the underlying food addiction. Simply put, there is *no chance of recovery* if the addiction is not recognized and treated. Cruelly, we will keep the food addict alive only to overeat again. Sadly, this was the case with Walter.

There are now a growing number of food addicts in the final stage of the disease. Many are extremely obese, unable to work, and, like Lawrence, have become virtual shut-ins. At the end, Lawrence became so obese that he was unable to get out of bed. Too embarrassed to call an emergency response team, he felt imprisoned in his bedroom. To get medical care, he had to rely on doctors like me who were willing to make home visits.

Could Walter or Lawrence have been served better if someone had been able to recognize sooner the telltale pattern of addiction that their behaviour exhibited instead of focusing on their obesity alone? I believe so. In the final chapter of this book, you will hear the success stories of people who have found a solution to their food addiction before it was too late. Once their addiction was addressed, the obesity often resolved itself.

It is unfortunate that misdiagnosis and under-diagnosis of food addiction is all too common for many of us who have sought help with our weight and food issues. The next chapter highlights this problem and its consequences. Food addiction is a shape-shifter, and, although food addiction has identifiable characteristics, it has as many different appearances as there are food addicts. It is easy to miss it — unless you are looking for it.

CHAPTER NINE

FOOD ADDICTION: THE GREAT SABOTEUR

Today the scientific evidence supporting a diagnosis of food addiction is mounting. Yet few among the obese or those suffering from eating disorders benefit from this breakthrough. Why is that diagnosis not more commonly recognized and given? Some experts, such as surgeon and TV personality Dr. Mehmet Oz, act as if they have never heard of the term. Others, such as Audrae Erickson, who, as former president of the Corn Refiners Association lobbied on behalf of corn sweeteners, criticize it mercilessly.[1]

What is most disturbing is that some eating disorder professionals agree that while addictions to some foods might exist, these are still best treated within the eating disorder framework of moderation and portion control.

Champions of this perspective are Dr. Phillip McGraw (better known as Dr. Phil), members of the International Association of Eating Disorders Professionals (IAEDP), and the writers of countless websites (LiveStrong.com, LoseIt.com, etc.) dedicated to helping people lose weight.[2] They believe that food addiction can be cured by learning to eat moderate portions, exercising more frequently, and dealing with the emotional factors they believe are at the root of all cravings to overeat. What they don't suggest is removing the triggering substances. Most commercial weight-loss programs know that people don't want to follow a plan that will eliminate their favourite "drug" — whether it's sugar, bread, or ice cream — if the message is to eliminate it … forever.

It is easy to understand why clinicians have been reluctant to acknowledge the dynamic of food addiction: it shows itself in many complex forms, truly a coat of many colours. Many food addicts are obese, but many are of normal weight; some are underweight. One study, which used the Yale Inventory of Food Addiction, estimated that 10 percent of underweight individuals are food addicts, as are 6 percent of those classified as normal weight and 14 percent of those who are overweight. The Yale Inventory also shows that 37 percent of the obese are food addicted (Meule *et al.*, 2011).[3] A 2015 review of the science posits a conservative 26 percent of the population. I suspect this is a low estimate.

To further complicate matters, in many cases people who are suffering from obesity also exhibit the emotional disturbances related to an eating disorder *and* the behaviours typical of food addiction. Even research aimed to tease out the distinctions between both conditions highlights their intermingling. A 2017 Australian study applying both the Binge Eating Scale and the Yale Food Addiction Scale found a significant overlap between binge eating and food addiction; both conditions showed high levels of depression, poor impulse control, and low self-esteem.[4] It is no wonder that obesity has been so difficult to treat effectively.

Missing the diagnosis of food addiction is especially dangerous in this already highly confusing area. Food addiction is often the hidden saboteur that is undermining an otherwise solid treatment program.

Clara's Story

Clara, who is in her late fifties, weighs more than six hundred pounds. Truthfully, though, this woman does not know her weight, because she has no access to a scale that could measure it.

For a long time, Clara was an excessive drinker, but because she was unable to control her drinking she has not touched a drop for more than a decade. It's interesting that she successfully quit alcohol even though her increasing girth made it impossible for her to leave home to attend the twelve-step meetings that had helped her achieve this. Recognizing that her consumption of food mirrored the familiar patterns she'd recognized with her drinking years earlier, she wanted to try a twelve-step program for her eating.

A local group of recovering food addicts, who were part of Overeaters Anonymous, heard about Clara's plight, and when they realized that she was having trouble detoxing, they offered to provide her with in-person support, twenty-four hours a day, for a full week. With their help, Clara became sugar and flour abstinent for the first time in her life. To her amazement, she realized that she had never felt so physically and emotionally good. But when her OA supporters left, Clara knew she was in a predicament.

Over the years, Clara's weight had made it impossible to get out shopping or even move easily around her house. She became dependent on her daughter, especially for food preparation. Her daughter did the cooking and agreed to prepare the foods on Clara's new food plan, but she also continued to cook her own favourite foods since she had no interest in abstaining from sugar and flour herself. The tantalizing smells filled the house each night, and foods that Clara was not supposed to eat were easily available around the kitchen. At first, Clara was able to push aside the desserts and baked goods, but easy access to the treats she had long enjoyed made resistance difficult. Eventually, Clara gave in and ate the forbidden foods.

Although no longer abstinent from sugar and flour, she stayed in contact with her OA community for more than a year. She tried half-heartedly to go back on the abstinent food plan, but she kept falling off the wagon. When it was apparent that she was not going to lose weight through dietary changes, her doctor recommended that she have bariatric surgery. She agreed, hoping that the surgery would give her the extra push she needed to get back on track.

Her surgeon, concerned that her weight would increase the risk of complications from the procedure, had her admitted to a ward at the hospital for a year. This ward supposedly specializes in treating food addiction. The idea was to stay on a medically restricted, low-calorie diet to lose weight. Clara was happy about this, but she became confused when the nutritionist at the bariatric clinic did not counsel her to abstain from sugar and flour or help Clara to stay abstinent while in the hospital. The ward kept giving her low-fat starchy foods that left her feeling hungry and dissatisfied. She spent time with the other morbidly obese patients in the ward, who also complained about their diets. Soon, they took to ordering out for pizza and other fast foods. After a year of living in this hospital, Clara actually *gained* weight and never qualified for bariatric surgery.

If that doesn't qualify as sabotage, I don't know what does.

Will's Story

Will, who was in his early thirties and tipped the scales at 380 pounds, wanted to lose weight. His health insurance provider and the professionals at his local hospital told him that his only option was a medically supervised weight-loss program. He willingly tried the program four times, and during each effort lost close to a hundred pounds. But he kept relapsing and would regain every pound of his lost weight.

Will resisted attending OA because, he said, the meetings had "no young people and no men." At that time, he did not know about FA (Food Addicts in Recovery Anonymous), another twelve-step program, which attracts a higher ratio of men than women. (Founded in 1998, FA uses the twelve-step model but emphasizes "allergies" to sugar and flour in addition to problems with portion control. Their diet eliminates all sugar and flour.)

His primary-care doctor suggested that he attend an in-patient program. While agreeable to this idea, Will could not find a program that had beds big enough to support his weight. Also, most of these programs offered treatment geared toward those with eating disorders, with a client base consisting primarily of young, female anorexics and bulimics, who were often underweight, or only moderately overweight.

Will received funding for a week-long residential workshop for food addicts, but this program presented a similar problem. The bathrooms at the retreat centre could not accommodate his size. Although he liked the program and managed to practise abstinence from the beginning, Will was too embarrassed to ask for help with using the toilet and shower, so he decided to leave against the staff's advice.

Clara and Will both need a kind of help that is unavailable to them. They represent the rapidly growing numbers of morbidly obese people. This segment of the population has needs that are especially dire, yet most services that are available are not accessible to them. Although only 3 to 4 percent of the U.S. population is in this category, that still represents almost twelve million people. If the exploding growth in childhood obesity, in particular, is not stopped, the number of morbidly obese in North America will continue to grow. We have no way to effectively treat the food addicts among them.

As I have already noted, the current solution for this group of people is bariatric surgery, which succeeds for 70 percent of patients (although the success rate drops to 40 percent after five years). Most people who are considered bariatric surgery "failures" demonstrate the symptoms of food addiction, although none were diagnosed as such. So, there are three to five million chronically ill, obese people with multiple secondary illnesses, for whom we have no workable answers.

Unfortunately, Clara and Will are not alone.

Tom's Story

Tom is an African-American man in his forties who has always had trouble controlling his weight. As an adult, he became an excellent math teacher and a loving father, but his weight problems dominated his life. He had to take high doses of blood pressure medication and was required to undergo weekly dialysis treatments that he dreaded. He began attending OA and soon came to accept that he was a food addict. Still, he kept relapsing. Tom heard about an extended food addiction treatment workshop where he could learn to become abstinent from sugar, flour, and binge foods, and he promptly signed up. Although most groups contained few other people of colour, the group he found himself in included three other African-Americans.

The program was a success. Tom was able to get the support he needed not only from the program itself, but also from these members. Together, he and the three other persons of colour discussed some incidents of racism in the group, leading to Tom realizing he'd never been angry in the presence of a white person before; he had been taught by his parents *not* to show anger when in the presence of white people. This insight made Tom feel empowered.

Although Tom felt that he had made some progress with the emotional issues stemming from the racism that he had experienced, he found that he was also angry at the effort he had had to expend in order to protect his recovery from food addiction. Why did people keep pushing him to eat foods that would lead to a relapse? In the group, he worked on being honest about his anger and dealing with it in less self-destructive ways.

Prior to this experience, Tom had felt left out in his twelve-step programs because the racism he experienced in his daily life was not addressed — it was seen as an "outside" issue that could unnecessarily derail the group's intent — and he found therapy unhelpful since its focus was not on food addiction. He also had trouble finding a therapist who understood the nuances of food addiction. Constantly, he felt that he had to choose between working through the unresolved emotions underlying his food addiction or finding a program to support abstinence from trigger foods. In truth, he needed both, since success relied on making progress on both issues. When Tom eventually found an extended-stay halfway house where he could get support for both his underlying emotional issues and his eating, his relapses finally stopped.

Late-stage food addicts like Tom often exhibit intense unresolved trauma. It would be easy to make a simple diagnosis of trauma-induced eating (that led to obesity), binge eating disorder, or bulimia for such individuals. But the underlying theme is obvious: food addiction exists as a dynamic that, when unaddressed, will undermine the best efforts of even the most determined person. Without addressing the addiction, treatment can actually make things worse.

I believe that food addicts need the same type of support offered to alcoholics and drug addicts. They need to detoxify first and then learn about their disease, while dealing with the thoughts and feelings that arise once they are off their drug. Quite often, psychological issues do not become obvious until food addicts have been abstinent for a long period of time. That's why ongoing support is needed to prevent addicts from relapsing in a panicky effort to cope.

There Is Hope!

The message of food addiction has been trumpeted in the popular press throughout the years. Among the supporters are:

- Dr. David A. Kessler, former head of the U.S. Food and Drug Administration and author of *The End of Overeating.*
- William Dufty, sixth husband of actress Gloria Swanson and the writer of 1975's *Sugar Blues,* which established the couple as two of the first anti-sugar advocates.
- Michael Prager, the former *Boston Globe* editor, who wrote the autobiography, *Fat Boy, Thin Man,* which is about his experience of being an extremely obese child who lost his weight and *kept it off* once he admitted he was a food addict.
- Rev. Margaret Bullitt-Jonas, the Missioner for Creation Care in the Diocese of Western Massachusetts and the author of *Holy Hunger: A Woman's Journey from Food Addiction to Spiritual Fulfillment.*
- Susan Peirce Thompson, of the *Bright Line Eating: The Science of Living Happy, Thin and Free* program. As a previous crack addict who found sugar addiction profoundly more isolating and embarrassing, Susan has designed a food plan and intensive program that calls for no sugar or flour. She also encourages social support via workshops and social media to prevent relapses back to the addictive eating.
- Judy Collins, who wrote *Cravings: How I Conquered Food,* which tells of her lifelong struggle with alcoholism and food addiction. It was not until she found a twelve-step peer support program in the community that focused on food

addiction that she was able to find peace with her weight and eating behaviour.

In each case, the writers tell of losing weight — the amounts range from ten to over a hundred pounds — only to regain all of it again. Most repeated the pattern several times before they understood what they were doing wrong. They would practise abstinence first and then move into the portion-control stage that typically follows. Once they ate their trigger foods again, the portions would get too difficult to contain and splurges became a daily phenomenon. Each became trapped in the vicious cycle of "yo-yo" dieting, which went on for years. Most had sought talk therapy, which did little to help their problems of overeating and weight gain. Only by treating themselves as addicts did they find sustainable recovery.

One convincing story among these personal testimonials is that of Jack LaLanne, one of television's first exercise gurus.[5] LaLanne's slim and muscular body has usually been attributed to his physical regimen; this was what promoted his exercise business, after all. But off-screen, he told a different story. He could not stop overeating. One day he read about Swanson and Dufty, who had maintained their weight loss only after they abstained from sugar and other refined foods. When LaLanne tried a similar approach, he discovered to his delight that his cravings disappeared. It turns out that the "exercise man" had to recover from food addiction *before* he could build a healthy body through exercise. The message: when a person suffering from food addiction finds suitable treatment, sustainable recovery is possible.

Pockets of research for the few food addiction programs that have existed show the same good news. A study of the residential food addiction treatment program offered by the now-defunct Glenbeigh Psychiatric Hospital of Tampa, Florida, found that by using an addiction model of treatment, the staff was able to report a success rate that any substance abuse program would envy.[6] Even better, the study illustrated that one-third of the patients continued to follow an abstinence-based food plan five years later *without* relapse. Another third occasionally relapsed, but were still able to reclaim recovery. These were the same clients who had, on average, attempted a dozen diets and two to three years of therapy without success prior to embracing a food addiction program.

Participants in a series of five-day residential workshops for food addicts showed comparable results. These sessions, modelled on the Glenbeigh process, are today facilitated by the staff at ACORN Food Dependency Recovery Services. ACORN is a Florida-based professional group of recovered food addicts who run workshops and support groups for people with eating issues. Of the 1,400 participants who have been surveyed, almost everyone who attended the workshops has been able to stop overeating while "protected" during their stay. Many of these had been unable to achieve anything like recovery through other methods.[7]

So, with adequate diagnosis and treatment, food addicts can thrive. This is my mission, the essential reason for writing this book.

There is one group whose issues with food are particularly difficult to treat. They suffer from the greatest of saboteurs: anorexia. Because overeating is the common symptom between bulimia and binge eating, these two conditions are most commonly confused with food addiction. It might seem odd, however, to envision the *aversion* to food typically seen in an anorexic as a manifestation of the same phenomenon. The following chapter will elucidate this possibility. Although I acknowledge that anorexia exists as an entity in its own right, I believe that there are many anorexics who may actually be disguised food addicts. Many anorexics simply do not respond to conventional treatment. I believe that if given the proper diagnosis, some of these "anorexics" can finally find relief from their painful condition. This is the subject of the next chapter.

CHAPTER TEN

FOR THE ANOREXIC

Ruthann's Story

Ruthann is a fifty-eight-year-old woman who has struggled with anorexia for more than forty years. Her weight has ranged from as low as seventy-seven pounds to, at its highest, one hundred and thirty-three pounds. She is five-foot-six and, as I sit looking at her in the library of her brownstone apartment in London, I'd estimate that right now she weighs approximately one hundred pounds. She is tiny, lean, and delicate, and although she has never been fat, she tells me emphatically that she feels she is fat right now.

I'm sitting on a couch draped with textiles that her daughter made, surrounded by books and paintings that her mother created. There are photos of her extended family nicely arranged on her walls. She is married to a successful man and she herself is the published author of a number of historical crime novels. She has worked as a writer for many of the years that she has lived in England.

When Ruthann was fourteen years old, the self-consciousness of puberty evolved into a loathing of her body. Like so many girls at that stage of their lives, she saw herself as fat and called herself "the pig." In an effort to cope with this self-image, she chose to go on a five-hundred-calorie-a-day diet. When she did not lose weight quickly enough, she started a regimen of doing over one thousand push-ups a day.

To motivate herself, she set a goal weight of 109 pounds. If she could attain that goal, she told herself, she would be happy.

One morning, she discovered that she weighed 107 pounds. Frowning, she realized she was still not happy, so she resolved to lose more weight until she felt happy. She thought that might be at the one-hundred-pound mark. Reducing her diet from a serving of cottage cheese a day to only one curd of cheese, she lost weight rapidly but did not feel any happier. At seventy-eight pounds, she ended up in the hospital, sick and depressed.

Medical personnel in the 1970s did not know what to do with her. Although the term *anorexia nervosa* had been around since the late nineteenth century, it was mainly a subject for a small cohort of specialists. (It wasn't until 1983, when pop singer Karen Carpenter died, that widespread media attention brought the disease to the mainstream.) Ruthann was put on the antipsychotic drug Stellazine and discharged under the care of a therapist. But her disease progressed when she discovered laxatives and purging. Before the end of the year, she was readmitted to hospital for laxative abuse. When she was released, the behaviour continued. Over the dinner table, her frustrated and frightened father would shout at her, "Eat this for your mother!" So Ruthann would eat, but later, purge the food. She developed a permanent scar on her hand from her teeth grating the skin during the repeated vomiting.

Ruthann's parents were survivors of the horrific Nazi extermination camps. Her father was a talented pianist who miraculously managed to save his life by attracting the attention of a German mentor who arranged for the precocious young man to be taken to safety. Later, her father became a successful concert musician who played in recital halls across Europe and America. As someone who had survived the Holocaust, he could not understand why Ruthann refused to eat; she looked like the poor prisoners suffering in the camps.

Ruthann's mother was also very talented. She was a painter and, like Ruthann's father, worked hard at her career. Both of her parents put the demands of their careers ahead of Ruthann's childhood needs. "All

I ever wanted was my mother's love," Ruthann confided to me. "I was starving for this."

To care for Ruthann, her parents sponsored a Dutch immigrant to act as her nanny. Unfortunately, she was not very maternal. When Ruthann cried and refused to eat, she strapped the child down and force-fed her. Ruthann remembers this as the time when she stopped eating and started to vomit. She was only four years old.

As the diagnosis of anorexia became more widely known, Ruthann received therapy to deal with her eating disorder. For more than twenty years, she went to a psychodynamic therapist four times a week, exploring the childhood and family dynamics that she believed contributed to her anorexia.

Apart from the disturbing relationship with her nanny, Ruthann also had difficult relations with her parents. To comfort her mother, she felt she had to fill in for her father's constant absences, and it seemed that her mother would withhold love from her while at the same time consulting with the little girl about her work and career issues. Once Ruthann told her: "I am only eleven years old! Let me *be* eleven years old." But most of the time she was too afraid to assert herself, worried that her mother, like her father, might become absent.

Ruthann also remembers her childhood as being full of grand figures: she met academics, musicians, artists, even politicians who would drop by for memorable dinners. She felt she had to prove herself worthy of such a heritage. As a child of Holocaust survivors, and knowing both her parents had lost family members during the war, she felt tremendous pressure to excel, since they were so accomplished and because they had only their daughter to carry their dreams and aspirations forward.

With treatment, Ruthann's illness improved, but the overall picture was bleak. Her anorexia morphed into bulimic episodes. She remembers sometimes bingeing and purging seven to eleven times a day. By the age of thirty-three, she had developed complications from both eating disorders — cardiac abnormalities, electrolyte imbalances, severe osteoporosis from the anorexia — as well as a gradual erosion of all her teeth from the bulimia. By forty, she'd had ten tooth implants.

Today, Ruthann continues to struggle, eating only about six hundred calories a day. For breakfast, she will have frozen yogurt, an apple, or an egg-white omelette; she eats a banana for lunch; then two or three small shrimp or a small piece of turkey at dinner. She says she doesn't get hungry, explaining that "eating less always helps in eating less." Yet, she contradicts herself, also admitting that most of the time she feels she is starving. Sometimes, in the middle of the night, her hunger will wake her up. Hearing the siren call of food, she told me, "I get up and forage like an animal, steal my daughter's Halloween candy. I feel terribly guilty about this." The next day, discouraged and full of shame, she goes to the gym and attempts to burn off hundreds of calories.

Her psychiatrist says that he no longer has ambitions to cure her. She still meets with him twice a week and takes a daily antidepressant. She credits this drug with having stopped her bulimic urges completely. "It really stabilized me. It saved my life."

While the antidepressant did not alter the anorexic symptoms, Ruthann was heartily relieved that the bulimia was under control. The bulimia was more disruptive than the anorexia, she explains, describing the bloated, swollen cheeks and the gassy cramps caused by the ongoing use of laxatives. She also hated the weakness that came with the vomiting: the electrolyte imbalances had made her so dizzy she was never sure she could manage to walk more than a block. And stairs! "Specific subway stops were memorable for me," she said, "which ones had stairs I had to climb." What really controlled her symptoms was the nurturing care that a previous psychiatrist provided. She "loved me like a mother," Ruthann told me, sighing. She encouraged Ruthann to eat, requesting that Ruthann come in daily so she could witness her drink a tin of Ensure. When Ruthann was going through a particularly hard time, she was especially nurturing. When that psychiatrist retired from her practice last year, Ruthann felt as if her "surrogate mother" had left her. She remains bereft today.

That particular psychiatrist also encouraged Ruthann to go to a twelve-step program, advising her, "Just don't tell the members of the group that your drug of choice is food, instead of alcohol." Ruthann was willing to try and, to her surprise, found the group extremely helpful.

Attending twelve-step meetings initially seemed odd, but she came to realize that for her, anorexia was like having an addiction. She was obsessed and constantly fighting the urge to restrict or purge. Going to meetings every day made her feel less and less isolated. She met people who understood what addiction was, who did not mind if she called for help in the middle of the night. They were there, she told me, whenever she needed them.

Were Ruthann to show up for a consultation today, she would immediately be diagnosed as suffering from anorexia nervosa. The treatment would involve therapy for her emotional eating, medication, and a food plan that was not restrictive in quality or quantity of food. While treatment has helped in curbing the bulimia and reducing Ruthann's anorexic behaviour — such as restricting her food to starvation levels — her condition continues to dominate her life on a daily basis. Could an undiagnosed food addiction be the unaddressed dynamic that is still sabotaging her recovery?

Jeff's Story

Jeff was in his thirties when I met him. A successful jockey in the thoroughbred racing world, he had a small frame, wiry and thin. Maintaining this physique, keeping a low weight, is necessary, he explained, because exceeding the weight limit at pre-race weigh-ins means disqualification. (Jockeys fear the scales they all must face before a race, which are known in their world as "the Oracle.") It's not surprising, then, that he and his colleagues weigh themselves daily and frequently binge and purge, abusing laxatives and diuretics. A 2008 study from England's Brunel University reported that "all jockeys embark on extreme programs to get their weight down, known as 'wasting.'" The study added: "this might involve a combination of starvation, deliberate dehydration, excessive sauna use and even self-induced vomiting, known colloquially as flipping."[1]

Jeff, like some other athletes and dancers, also used cocaine to control his weight, but over time he found that he could not manage his cocaine use. After he was caught snorting a line just before a race, he was ordered to enter a residential treatment program; if he did not, he was told he would lose his job. But each time he stopped using cocaine, he rediscovered a voracious appetite that had him eating uncontrollably. Although he knew that using drugs could cost him his career, in the end, he preferred a cocaine addiction to the consequences of his lack of control over food.

I didn't believe Jeff suffered from an eating disorder; I think he suffered from an addiction, which included cocaine as well as food. Why? Like Ruthann, who was addicted to food as well as having an eating disorder, Jeff consumed food in a manner that closely resembled his abuse of drugs. I felt that if we addressed his addiction first — whether it be food or cocaine -- the other issues would sort themselves out later, but this was not to be. After he discontinued our therapeutic sessions, I don't believe he was successful at sobriety.

Food Addiction: A Coat of Many Colours

While food addicts may be suffering from emotional distress, they are experiencing a phenomenon that is distinctly different from that which drives a normal eater who eats too much or someone with an eating disorder. Food addicts are chemically dependent on specific foods. The main problem is not the behaviour or the feelings that need to be self-medicated, although each might be a factor in the background. After all, who doesn't want to eat chocolate when they are depressed? Food soothes and comforts unruly emotions.

Nor is food addiction about weight. Although most are overweight, many food addicts are normal weight or even underweight. There are few studies of food addiction, but based on my own clinical experience and a study by Yale University's Rudd Center for Obesity Research and Policy, I estimate that as much as 50 percent of the obese, 20 to 30 percent of the overweight, and up to 10 percent of the normal weight people are food addicted. I also believe about 10 percent of those who are underweight may also be food addicted.

Food addiction is a chemical dependency related to specific food ingredients. The food addict's response to food is biochemically different from that of a normal eater or an emotional eater. For food addicts, it is the physical effects of food, not the emotional ones, that initially drive the cravings. Emotions are often a trigger to start eating, but, once triggered by the food, the phenomenon of a craving, or obsession, to eat becomes larger than the emotion needing to be placated.

As the disease of addiction progresses, food addicts become powerless over their physical cravings for some foods — especially sugar, flour, grains, fat, salt, and caffeine — just as alcoholics are predisposed to being chemically dependent on alcohol and drug addicts to heroin, cocaine, or prescription drugs. As well as arising from a specific food, addiction can also be triggered by an excess volume of any food. When a person exceeds what we might call "normal" eating, the hormonal checks and balances of hunger and satiety are lost. Sometimes just the act of eating — the munching and crunching of food in the mouth — provides so much comfort and pleasure that the person can't stop. Some food addiction twelve-step groups ask their members to weigh and measure their food because some people can binge on bag after bag of carrots. (People who exhibit this behaviour are known as "volume addicts.")

If we reconsider Ruthann's story, we can see an emerging pattern of addictive behaviour around food. She craves food to the point where she cannot have any of it in the house, not even flour. She grinned ruefully as she told me about her relationship to flour. "Flour, water, salt, and garlic equals garlic pancakes." And that meant unbearable cravings and voracious binges on pancakes — until all the flour was consumed — often in the middle of the night. Discussing her relationship to food overall, Ruthann told me: "If I could live on desserts, I would want only desserts. But if I eat them, I just want more and more. I love sugar. If I don't have it, I will go into shock, I crash…. Once I start the sugar, that is all I want."

Bulimorexia: The Norton's Center for Eating Disorders and Obesity

Psychologist and author Renae Norton, who founded Cincinnati's Norton Center for Eating Disorders and Obesity, has worked with many anorexics and bulimics throughout her career. Over the past few years, she explained to me in a telephone interview, she has witnessed an alarming trend. "Young women who were being treated for their eating disorders, especially the anorexics, are now developing bulimorexia," she said, a phenomenon where the separate conditions of anorexia and bulimia merge to become a single, even more difficult disease to treat.

This condition is often caused because anorexics go into a residential treatment setting where clinicians are intent on making them gain weight. The staff feed these clients foods that are highly palatable and intended to create weight gain. These foods are high in fat and carbohydrates. The starved anorexics typically gain twenty pounds in their first twenty days of treatment.

However, Norton thinks the patients, once discharged, leave worse than when they first came into treatment. Arriving with symptoms specific to anorexia, they leave in the confused mental state which Norton has defined as bulimorexia: the patient's appetite for sugar and carbs is voracious, yet she is determined to lose the weight she has just gained at any cost. These individuals are much more likely to die, asserts Norton, because after treatment their bingeing or purging often escalates to lethal levels. They crave food more than ever before, yet they are equally determined to lose the weight gained in the hospital.

Norton meets her patients after they have tried the traditional routes of therapy for anorexics and are now in this muddle of both conditions. Typically, though, by the time she sees them, the disease is extremely volatile. She works hard with them, but she acknowledges that their response to treatment is less favourable than those who suffer from either condition alone. There is also a much higher rate of relapse.

According to Norton, this mixed condition is more common than we think. In her online survey of people suffering from eating disorders, she found that 38 percent identified as having bulimorexia. This is in contrast to those who identified themselves as specifically anorexic (25 percent), bulimic (12 percent), and emotional eaters (almost 11 percent). Of the people who responded to her survey, only 13 percent identified as obese.[2]

Norton is convinced that the root cause of this disorder is the introduction of the "addictive foods" into the treatment diet provided for eating disorders. She believes that a diet rich in sugar, starch, and fat, which is typical of what an eating disorder program would serve, is toxic to the highly vulnerable brains of anorexics and bulimics. I agree. Anorexics who have starved themselves for days, or bulimics who have become dependent on sugar and other rich foods, are vulnerable to the high caloric diet — especially menu items heavy on high fructose corn syrup, the basis of most fattening foods. Their brains are especially sensitive to this heightened neurochemical mixture; for these patients, the reward value of these foods is considerably higher than it would be for a person who has not become either dependent on sugar or deficient in it due to an eating disorder. That high reward value is what tips the balance — now the person not only has an eating disorder, but also a food addiction.

Anorexia, Bulimorexia, and Food Addiction

How does this addiction happen? Acute stress, which could be caused by a potential illness or a sudden loss of income, sparks a burst of dopamine in the reward centre of the brain, presumably to prompt us into action so we can deal with the oncoming crisis. This explains why some of us are "crisis junkies," thriving on the dopamine pumping in our system when we are anxious. The starving state that is typical of an anorexic or bulimorexic creates its own kind of stress. This is intentional; the brain provides an increased dopamine gush to spur us to forage for food. Our pulse quickens. The anticipation of food is so heightened that the smell, even the promise, of food makes us salivate and powerfully desire it. The hungrier we are, the more the taste of food will intensify. This is the reason why any food seems more delicious when we are extremely hungry.

The anorexic is the quintessential hungry hunter, poised in search of food, basking in the anticipatory dopamine rush of food soon to come. This exciting feeling *stops* the moment the anorexic takes her first bite. Certainly, the first few bites of food will give exquisite pleasure — the brain, after all, has been primed for it. But with each bite, the anticipation and pleasure ebb. The anorexic, accustomed to this type of high, becomes more "sober" the more they've eaten. Most anorexics say they feel *better* when they are hungry. They are not lying. Anorexics truly feel a high, even if they are near death.

Purging can also become addictive. The bulimic experiences a complex string of neurochemical and biochemical events. The vomiting process itself induces pain, so that the bulimic feels a release of opiates that numbs emotional pain and creates the good feeling of being "cleansed." Vomiting also impairs the response of leptin, a hormone that plays a key role in regulating appetite. Recall that leptin, which creates a sense of fullness and satiety, is released about thirty minutes after eating. When the bulimic eats and purges, leptin is unable to have its assuaging effect, and so there is no feeling of fullness and satiety that will halt the eating. Dopamine and endorphins, sparked by the sugary and fatty foods typical of a binge, mount with each binge/purge cycle, creating euphoria without end.

An appreciation of this addiction dynamic is crucial for a food addict's recovery. While an eating disorder may aptly explain anorexic and bulimic symptoms, it is just as likely that the eating disorder is part of the addictive disorder itself. It may not be principally the result of deep-seated emotional issues. If the person is a food addict, rather than someone suffering from a true eating disorder, then the typical treatment used for eating disorders is not helpful. As Norton has found with her bulimorexic clients, that treatment can actually be dangerous. A modified food plan based on our North American food pyramid (changed to a food plate in 2011) may inadvertently undermine the recovery of a person who appears to be an anorexic or bulimic but is, in fact, a food addict. Could this be the reason for the high rate of recidivism for eating disorders?[3]

Ruthann's psychiatrist observed that Ruthann was not responding well to treatment. Seeing an addictive dynamic in Ruthann's eating behaviour, she intuitively suggested the AA program. Ruthann readily admitted that she felt "addicted" to her behaviours around food and recognized that feeling when she binged *and* when she restricted her food. "If I eat a certain amount," she said, "I wonder if I can cut that in half and then in half again and then in half again."

How little she can eat, paradoxically, is never enough.

When Ruthann was undergoing treatment, food addiction had not yet been accepted as a viable diagnosis in the clinical trade journals that govern the standard of practice that her psychiatrist was expected to follow. So, she insisted that Ruthann eat a diet that focused on weight gain and emotional health, rather than on determining what foods could be triggering her relapses. As a medical practitioner, the psychiatrist diligently followed the protocols available to her: medicating with the use of an antidepressant, prescribing regular therapy, and insisting that Ruthann follow a healthy eating regimen that consisted of fruits, dairy, proteins, and low-fat foods. But the fact that she also recommended a twelve-step program for Ruthann was frankly progressive and placed her outside the norm of standardized treatment.

Presenting a treatment plan that addresses both an eating disorder *and* a food addiction (which Ruthann very likely demonstrates) presents a challenge. I would suggest that if it becomes apparent that the typical eating-disorder meal plan, which includes moderation of trigger foods, results in persistent relapses to bingeing or restrictive behaviour, a food addiction plan should be attempted. This would involve removing trigger foods, especially sugar and flour, *and* weighing food portions — so that neither bingeing nor restricting can occur. This meal intervention should be done under the watchful eye of a clinician or food buddy. Close attention to both eating dynamics may be crucial to success for these complicated eating syndromes.

Food addiction could be the missing piece to the puzzle of the recidivism that commonly occurs after even intensive treatment for eating disorders. Food addicts of all varieties need to remove the addictive foods and behaviours from their diet in order to obtain any hope for long-term food sobriety and serenity.

CHAPTER ELEVEN

HITTING BOTTOM: I NEED HELP!

The "moment of lucidity" is when addicts decide it is time to get off the bus that is hurtling toward their own destruction — the moment when people struggling with addiction decide that the pain of using their drug *outweighs* the pain of trying to stop using it. How will you know when you have hit your bottom? How bad does it have to get?

Surprisingly, many addicts long for this moment to occur. They keep using, but at the same time hope that they will finally get it, they will finally find the motivation, the control — the *something* that will propel them to change their behaviour. What is this magical moment that some describe as a spiritual awakening? What does it look like for a food addict?

The moment of clarity is different for everyone. For one person, it might be when he no longer can be weighed at the hospital because there is no scale that registers higher than 350 pounds. At that moment, he refuses to live with the shame any longer. For another person, it's the moment when she realizes that her partner is no longer willing to live with her binge-induced mood swings and lack of sex drive. Many addicts may never find their bottom, and, as we have seen with Lawrence and Walter in earlier chapters, they will remain prisoners of their addiction until death takes them.

So, for those who do find their bottom, how bad did it have to get? Here are our own personal stories, showing how unique and powerful each bottom can be.

Vera's Story

It was a busy morning at the Amherstburg nursing home. I was eighteen years old and working at my first "real" job. I had taken the job relishing the idea of working with older people and I was determined to make a good impression. On this particular day, though, I was already running behind schedule. With only fifteen minutes left before the kitchen staff rang for the empty trays, I still had eight more residents to feed. Unsure that I could finish in time, I darted from one bed to the next, trying to get each patient to chew and swallow. In the end, I gave up any serious attempt to be gentle and began stuffing food in each person's mouth. I knew this wasn't good care, but I could not fathom how the other nursing aides got this job done in a more compassionate manner.

With lunchtime finished and all the residents' faces scrubbed, I was exhausted, although I knew that in no time dinner would be ready and the whole process would start again. My shift seemed to be an endlessly frantic process of feeding, washing up, and then feeding again.

One day, after rushing through another meal, I discovered that a number of trays returned to the trolley contained meals that appeared to have been barely touched. I tasted some of the cold beef and mashed potatoes. It wasn't bad, and it seemed foolish to waste food. Often, my own fridge was bare — I seldom shopped and I did not like to cook. In those days, I was mainly living on sub sandwiches, burgers and fries, chips and chocolate bars. Often, I would just smoke a cigarette to take away the edge of hunger.

Gradually, I began eating my meals from the patients' trays — at first only taking food that looked untouched, but later consuming anything that looked edible. I especially liked the small desserts: the apple crumble, custard, or biscuits and jellies. These treats were often still warm and were usually untouched since I had had to rush away the plates to get them on the trolley before the slow eaters could finish their meals. I relished the desserts as little boosts of pleasure to get me through the long, stressful workday.

I was fairly sure the patients didn't miss them. The fact that I was stealing from someone's plate did occur to me, but I quickly rationalized it. They didn't know what was happening, I thought, and why shouldn't someone be enjoying this food? Why push dessert down someone's throat when she could barely finish the main course?

Then I met Mrs. Graham. An octogenarian with dementia, her head lolled back and her mouth caved into her face. Whenever I brought a forkful of food to her mouth, she groaned and swatted her hands at me. At the time, I saw her as just another wearisome patient in a sea of old faces. One day, when I was anxious, irritated, and hungry, we did not even finish her meal of green beans and roast beef before I began nibbling on her dessert. She ate so slowly she would never get to it, so, I thought, why wait? As I ate her peach tart, her eyes suddenly snapped open, narrowed, and focused on me. I could hear her mutter something. As our eyes locked, I saw, in that moment at least, she was no longer an incoherent geriatric. There she was, defenseless, bound, and propped up in her chair, yet aware of everything going on around her. She was, in that moment, an indignant person rightfully condemning my theft.

My face flushed with embarrassment. "Do you want another dessert?" I coughed. She glared at me without responding. She had not spoken for years, what did I expect now? A moment later, I left the room. Two weeks later I quit that job.

My second job was as manager of a small variety store in Windsor, Ontario. I lived rent-free in an apartment at the back of the store. It was a perfect job to fill my summer between finishing high school and starting university. My duties were to open the store at 8 a.m. and keep watch over the till until 11 p.m., when I locked up. The store was on a deserted side street in a working-class part of town, so sometimes I didn't see a customer for hours.

My favourite part of the job was ordering the stock. It was not difficult, as the only items the store regularly sold were chips, soda, cigarettes, and

candy. I especially liked to order the candy: I would pore over the cata-
logues, marveling at all the different colours, shapes, and tastes, knowing
that when they arrived I would treat myself to "samples." These treats
helped me get through the stifling boredom of the job, the long days of
silence in an often-empty store.

After closing up, I would walk through the store to my apartment in
the back. There I would drink or smoke pot until I fell asleep. Sometimes,
when I was high and hungry with the "munchies," I would remember drooling over the pictures in the order book, unpacking the boxes,
stacking the products in the front aisles, and so I'd fantasize about these
candies again.

One night, I decided that I had had enough of the fantasy. Without
turning on the light in the store, I crawled into the shop on my hands and
knees so no one on the street would see me through the front windows.
Then I filled my pockets with handfuls of jujubes, caramels, and bubble-
gum. Delectables! I was thrilled to know I would taste them all.

Somehow, I rationalized my theft — because it was night and I was on
my knees, I did not have to pay for these treats. In fact, I did not see this
as stealing at all. I was underpaid, working fifteen-hour days for only a
few hundred dollars a week, so I was just evening the score. The manager
never found out about these nightly raids and, by the age of twenty, I had
become a practiced thief.

One of my last jobs before I became serious about studying medicine
was working as a chambermaid at a hotel in London, England. By this
time in my life, I had given up trying to be thin. I was in my midtwenties
and had been struggling with my weight for more than five years. I had
already decided I would allow myself to eat whatever I wanted, whenever
I wanted, and as much as I wanted. I was overweight anyway; how much
worse could it get?

One of my daily chores at this hotel was delivering coffee and croissants each morning to our guests. Most of the chambermaids would eat
any croissants left over after preparing the guest trays. At first, I tried not
to eat them, since I was usually too bloated from a binge the night before.

I always finished my allotted rooms first and then waited for the
others to join me in the pantry. There I sat with the stacked trays from

the morning filled with half-eaten and uneaten croissants. This proved dangerous. The cold and greasy pastries would beckon and I would give in and start to nibble. I tried to resist, but I kept giving in. When there were no croissants left, I found myself still wanting more. Why did that keep happening? Rummaging through the garbage, I knew I would find something I could eat in there, always looking to make sure no one saw me. I was simultaneously horrified by this behaviour and blasé about it.

Once, when I was cleaning the room of a Turkish family, I discovered an open box of delicacies from an elite food store. I ate one, pretending that the box was meant to be garbage. Then I found another small box of candy of a type I had never seen before — large, powdery cubes filled with sweet, purple jelly. I decided to take just a bite of one. Then I picked up a full square and ate it, followed by another. It was delicious.

Had this been money or an article of clothing, I would have recognized it as stealing, and I did not steal from our guests. But this was just food. Yes, it was expensive food from a high-end confectionary, yet somehow I didn't see it as theft. In my mind, taking food was not like taking clothes or jewelry or, worse, money. Each day that I cleaned this room, I searched for another box of candy or exotic delight. Sometimes I rummaged in the closets, even in the luggage. These guests seemed to be hunting for unusual sweets and I was curious about everything they selected. When they left, it did not surprise me that I did not receive a tip. Deep down, I was just grateful they had not reported me.

For me, hitting bottom was not dramatic. It did not occur the night I sat for hours in an emergency department begging to be admitted so that I would not have to face myself alone in my empty apartment. Facing the terror of being alone with that insatiable hunger that led me to eat and eat and eat. That was not yet the bottom. Nor did it occur after the evening that I spent with the "Moonies," followers of the Unification Church who frequently hosted evenings targeted to recruit lonely people. I was so fearful to be alone with my addictive eating that I allowed myself to play silly games like musical chairs, intended to break the ice with strangers.

The experience of playing a child's game with a group of people I'd never met was humiliating, but it was better than trying to fight the demons of my food addiction. I hadn't hit bottom yet, but after this mortification I resolved to find better diversions to escape my relentless bingeing.

My fear of being alone with myself late at night resulted in extremes that shamed me. It also struck me as peculiar, since I had always prided myself on being ruggedly independent. No matter how well the day had gone, though, by evening I would get the same panicky feelings and, before I knew it, my hands trembled, my heart raced, and I experienced an incredible rush of excitement, flushed at the prospect of eating all of my forbidden goodies. My resolve not to binge dissipated with this potent combination of dread and excitement.

I could easily eat two full bags of groceries in one night — peanut butter, French bread, cottage cheese, chocolates, doughnuts, bagels, and croissants with Nutella or cream cheese. Then, stuffed and miserable, my belly cramping with gas, I would find it difficult to breathe. Feeling wretched, I would slink to the washroom for relief. The toilet bowl initially soothed me, the porcelain rim cool against my sweaty, bloated face. After vomiting, I cried and held the bowl tight, praying that each binge was the last for the night. But after the relief would come relentless thoughts of food again, taunting me. *What else can I eat? What have I not tried? What is still appealing? What could I still eat?*

Even while I cried, wanting it to stop, the excitement for more fruit-flavoured yogurt or ice cream or candy took over. Eventually, my mouth became raw, my tongue burned, my jaws ached, and my stomach muscles grew sore from the heaving purges. I felt drunk, puffy, and numb. Each night ended after eight or ten of these cycles. I would crawl into bed, sometimes at daybreak, filled with disgust and the resolve to quit. Yet, even this was not my bottom.

One night I hosted a party. Food addiction is all about strategies, and I had developed one for parties: If I drank a "moderate" amount of alcohol and then ate a "moderate" amount, I could get through an evening without overdoing it on either. It was the perfect compromise between my need to soothe myself with food and alcohol and my need to stave off the consequences of being too drunk or too caught up in a bulimic cycle. On this particular evening, I had already drunk my share of alcohol for the night and I was feeling pretty loud and boisterous.

The party was in full swing, so I put down my martini glass and headed for the buffet. I stuffed myself with all the tasty items people had brought, knowing that I would soon slip downstairs to the basement laundry room where I would vomit. I expected I would do that a few times over the course of the evening. This was my pattern: four double-double drinks and four binge-purge cycles usually got me through a party night.

Later, downstairs trying to throw up food, I was in a panic. I just couldn't quickly purge and I did not want to be away from the party for too long. What could I say if people noticed I had disappeared? I heaved and heaved, jabbed my fingers to the back of my throat, only grateful that the basement door was locked and the noise of the dancing and shouting upstairs hid the sound of my efforts to vomit. I started to whimper aloud with frustration.

"What's wrong?"

Mortified, I turned and saw an old friend staring at me with a mixture of confusion, disbelief, and concern. "How did you get in here?" I sputtered with a raspy voice. At first I was more embarrassed than I had ever felt before, then I lashed out. "This isn't what you think!"

He nervously explained that my partner had given him the keys to the basement so he could get more ice for the drinks from our deep freeze. "This isn't what you think," I repeated. My eyes dropped. I could not look directly at him. The shame was too overpowering.

Over the next few months, my friend and I drifted apart. I kept wanting to call, to explain, to make it right somehow, but I was stymied. What could I say? Perhaps the waning of interests that can occur between two old friends would have happened anyway, but my feeling of mortification at that moment when he found me retching into the laundry tub was enough for me. I was not going to experience such degradation and self-loathing again. I had finally reached my bottom.

Phil's Story

Maude Lapsley was a good woman. Intelligent, capable, and strong, she was beautiful and had a big heart. When she was twenty-four, her husband died, leaving her with four young children to take care of by herself. Maude immediately got herself a job as an assistant kindergarten teacher. She had her own children come to her classroom after school so they could do their homework while she prepared for the next day. During her first years as a single mother, she also went to school during the summer, working toward a college degree. With her certification in hand, she went on to become a popular first grade teacher, one in demand by parents who wanted her to teach their children to read.

But Maude's life had a dark side: her relationship with food. She kept gaining weight and, though this never seemed to affect her work, her commitment to her own children, or her generally good humour, it did affect her health. She dieted constantly, but she would gain back the weight almost as soon as she lost it. In her thirties, she developed severe high blood pressure and was put on medication. In her forties, her body began to show the physical effects of carrying so much extra weight: she would be out of breath after walking up a flight of stairs and her joints constantly ached. Her doctor kept giving her the latest diet advice, but, although she tried to follow his advice, it seemed she just had to have her sweets. "I can't give up those," she would say. After each failed attempt, she silently and guiltily berated herself.

At fifty-two, Maude Lapsley died suddenly of a massive heart attack. Her major goal that summer had been to lose fifty pounds on her latest diet. (Her doctor recommended that she eat only rice and drink lots of orange juice.) The official cause of death was listed as arterial thrombosis, but the more likely truth is that Maude Lapsley died of food addiction.

Maude was my grandmother. She died when I was four years old, and my mother and I cried for weeks. The real tragedy is that if she had known then what I know now, she could have been saved years of pain and misery and, probably, a needlessly early death.

Thirty years after her passing, I was having the same trouble with my weight as my grandmother had experienced. I kept losing it then immediately putting it back on. I even suffered a heart attack myself. But I could not leave food alone.

Even as a preschooler I showed signs of addiction. I stole food. I stole money to buy food. I obsessed about food. I gave directions by using restaurants and grocery stores as landmarks. I ate compulsively and I ate fast. At the dinner table, my parents would insist that I slow down, but as hard as I tried I would be done when they were still on their first couple of bites.

I binged on my grandmother's candy, drank Karo syrup out of the bottle, and ate brown sugar out of the box. I would toast slices of Wonder Bread with loads of butter and cinnamon, but I ate them faster than I could toast them.

And I told no one about what I was doing. I later understood that this secrecy allowed me to protect my "stash." I had already learned to always keep a private supply of food around so that I would never find myself without food late at night, after the stores were closed.

During high school, I was an active athlete, and spent two to four hours a day playing basketball and other sports. After a series of accidents in my senior year, though, I could no longer play sports. This change in my lifestyle happened around the same time that I went off to college and left behind my structured home life — and home cooking. It was at this time that I began gaining serious weight.

Through most of my freshman year at college, I wore a full-length overcoat all the time. I used to think, *I'm cool, man.* The truth, though, was that I was just trying not to look fat. By then I also had started trying diets, often by skipping breakfast, lunch, or dinner, or sometimes two or more of these a day. I counted calories. I ate "health food" and checked my menus with Adelle Davis, a nutritionist and author of *Let's Eat Right to Keep Fit.*[1] I could lose twenty-five to fifty pounds per diet, but I always gained it back.

By the time I finished graduate school I had become an obsessive dieter. From the outside, my career and my life looked successful. I had graduate degrees, a professorship, and a stellar resume. I had written books, was married with children, and I was a community activist.[2] Still, I was miserable. I had tried everything: vegetarianism, the all-liquor diet (which showed me I had another addiction), the rice diet, the Stillman diet, Hindu purification rituals, jogging, the exchange diet, fasting for two or three weeks at a time…. Nothing worked.

When it occurred to me that I needed to deal with my emotional issues to get the food under control, I tried a long list of other options: encounter groups, behavioural therapy, Eastern religion, yoga, co-counselling, Erhard Seminars Training, and The Forum. I even became a therapist and did graduate-level work setting up a program to help people learn how to control their eating. I acquired the sixty-six credits, the degree, and twenty-five pounds!

When I saw my doctor, he told me that my cholesterol and blood pressure were so high that I was a candidate for a heart attack. Instead of listening to my doctor's advice, I just stopped going to the doctor. A few years later, I went to a restaurant and asked for "the biggest item on the menu." Afterward, I suffered a heart attack. Despite that, I still refused to get help or even call 911 because I did not want to be put in the hospital and miss out on a banquet I was to attend the next day. I relaxed by breathing through the anxiety of that attack, thankfully mild, and woke up the next day thinking about how absolutely crazy my behaviour had been.

Years later, someone suggested I get tested for food allergies. After that, I abstained from all wheat for nineteen days. Then I sat down with a big plate of spaghetti and a loaf of bread I had made especially for the occasion. I was only about a fifth of the way into the spaghetti when I felt a funny sensation in my chest. I called to my then-wife, but before she could get downstairs, I had fallen on the floor. Thankfully, she kept me from going into shock.

I believe, although it was never confirmed, that I had almost gone into insulin shock. My body had a clear, unmistakable reaction to the wheat, so I now knew what was wrong with me, but I still could not stop eating wheat. Every day I would have a plan to avoid it, but by the end of the day I would have eaten a sandwich or some other form of wheat.

No matter how hard I tried, no matter what I did, I could not stop eating these foods for even one day. I felt completely demoralized and hopeless. I had identified the problem but lacked the will to solve it.

I truly thought this would be the end of my life and finally I shared this feeling at a men's support group I had joined, crying the whole time. Bless their hearts, the guys let me cry. Then, something wonderful happened. One of the men, a recovering alcoholic, said, "You eat just like I used to drink!"

This fellow's words changed my life. That's when I accepted that I was a food addict. That was my bottom.

Each addict reaches a different bottom. Some may seem undramatic — catching a glimpse in a mirror of oneself wolfing down a doughnut or other forbidden food, or staring fixedly at the scale — while others may be as climatic as mine or Phil's. Either way, it's at the moment of hitting bottom that there's also a chance of self-discovery and recovery.

CHAPTER TWELVE

WHAT DO I DO NOW?

Alexander looked at the bariatric surgeon in disbelief. "I have to wait how many years?" he sputtered. He had just recovered from his excitement at learning that, as a Canadian, he qualified for provincial funding that would allow him to get gastric banding surgery — a procedure that places an adjustable silicone band around the stomach. Now he'd been told that the waiting list was six to ten years long. *I'll be dead by the time my name comes up,* thought Alexander.

Six feet tall and four hundred pounds, Alexander was already suffering from diabetes and hypertension. He needed to reduce his weight. Gastric banding surgery had seemed the answer. If he had to wait for years to receive it, however, it might be too late. Unwilling to wait for provincial funding, he decided he would come up with the $16,000 himself to pay for the service privately. It took some doing, but he raised the money. That was in January 2008.

Alexander had already been through the diet mill. In his fifties, he was unwilling to go that route again. He had tried the low-fat diet, Weight Watchers, the Atkins Diet, and the low-glycemic diet, but they had all been failures in the end. He had tried medications. He even went to therapy to uncover the traumatic issues in his past that led to his weight problems. There, he came to understand how he had used food to "reward" himself so that he could tolerate the abuses he had been exposed to throughout his childhood. This insight was revealing, but like all the other ventures he tried, did not make his food cravings go away.

Even though he lost weight on his many diets — sometimes as much as one hundred pounds — the weight would eventually climb back, along with an additional fifty pounds. "Why do I keep doing this?" he asked himself in frustration.

When he found out that his provincial government plan might cover laparoscopic surgery, he decided to give it a try. He knew that he would have to change his diet again, but he felt confident that the surgery would boost his morale. Then he found out about the long waiting lists.

Since he was paying for it himself, Alexander could have chosen to get a gastric bypass, but he preferred the lap-band, done at a local cosmetic surgery clinic, as it was more affordable and required less recovery time afterwards. The lap-band is essentially a hollow tube filled with fluid that wraps around the stomach. When filled up, it constricts the stomach from the normal fist size to a small pouch, leaving little room for solid food. This makes it almost impossible to overeat or binge on typical junk foods. Alexander would be able to adjust the level of constriction according to how small he wanted his stomach to shrink; the smaller his stomach, the less food he would be able to ingest.

The surgery was a success. Alexander was discharged the next day with a diet plan in hand. Over the course of the next few months, he returned to the clinic a number of times, getting the lap-band adjusted to the most constricted level possible. This meant that he was only able to consume a liquid diet of soup and Jell-O. Although he was able to gradually include other foods, his portion sizes were always very minimal.

By the three-month mark, his typical meal plan included a protein powder drink in the morning, a small yogurt for lunch, and a can of tomato and beans for dinner. Alexander insisted this meagre diet was sufficient; he was eating whatever he wanted and as much as he needed. He never felt hungry. His weight dropped from 420 to 190 pounds. The staff at his surgeon's office were so impressed that they wanted to take before-and-after pictures to advertise their procedure. Alexander refused, explaining, "I have to see if I can keep it off." Losing weight was nothing new; keeping it off was the true test.

Two years later, Alexander started to eat a little bit of ice cream. It was just a small serving here and there, because he didn't want to gain weight again, but he'd decided he wanted to be able to eat *anything*, relying on portion size to keep his caloric load down. He knew this was risky. Other members of his family, having also undergone the surgery, barely changed their diets. Not surprisingly, they all gained back their weight afterward. Alexander sought help from the clinic about how to eat "normally," in a safe manner, but was dismayed to see that there was no aftercare offered. Beyond the instructions of how to eat in the recovery phase, there was neither guidance on how to maintain a healthy food plan, nor support when his food cravings returned.

Things went from bad to worse. Later that year, Alexander started to feel nauseous whenever he ate. He had a prior history of acid reflux and a hiatus hernia, so he wondered whether these were acting up again. Instead, investigations revealed Barrett's esophagitis — an inflammation of the esophagus that could lead to cancer if left untreated — was causing the discomfort in his chest whenever he ate.

No one could tell him whether his condition was caused by the lap-band procedure or had been brewing before it, but the treatment was clear. He had to have his stomach released from its constricted lap-band stranglehold. Three years later, Alexander's weight hit 420 pounds.

He cried the day he realized his weight was going up. He had already been struggling to control his appetite, which had returned with a resilience that horrified him. His cravings were relentless. Once again, he sought help from the clinic.

"I had no dietary advice or support," he told me bitterly. The clinic took no responsibility for any of the complications that arose after the procedure. Alexander felt he had been "ripped off" by a charlatan surgeon, talked into purchasing an expensive procedure that was supposed to be a cure but was really just a temporary solution. No one informed him of what he now knows in hindsight: Obesity is a chronic disease for which there is *no* guaranteed cure.

"It's a scam," he concluded. When he heard that the clinic had been forced to close down one year after his surgery, he was not surprised. Alexander conceded that there probably are well-intentioned surgeons who do good work, but he remains suspicious of the surgeries performed in cosmetic surgery clinics. (lap-band surgery is more often performed in clinics than by surgeons in hospitals, but standards and regulations governing this relatively new phenomenon are still evolving.)

Now Alexander had yet another failure to add to his list of aborted attempts to lose weight, with no hope in sight. All he has been able to find in Nova Scotia, where he moved in 2014, was a partially funded government program that offers Nutrisystem as its foundation. It consists of a ten-week regimen that offers a "sugared milk food replacement fast," along with a year of group education and sharing. He was not interested in this short-term approach.

He had not heard about food addiction until we met in April 2013. Now, convinced that food addiction is his problem, Alexander is trying to create the social supports he needs in his rural community in Nova Scotia, since services of this kind are uncommon outside major urban centres. While professionals do seem to be aware of food addiction research, it is never the focus in any of their programs.

Since we met, Alexander, with the help of his wife, has been able to get his weight down to 300 pounds. He wants to lose more as he is still uncomfortable with his body and continues to struggle with food cravings. But he feels defeated, even while acknowledging that he needs to face his addiction rather than "default to early death and disability."

My last contact with him was a hopeful email he sent me just before Christmas 2017. He expected to undergo a vertical sleeve gastrectomy in the new year and is now following the pre-operative diet he has been given. He wrote, "In the past, I have proven to be very good at following these regimens; the challenge begins months afterwards when they are completed." He assured me that his knowledge of which foods to avoid would inform his transition from the post-operative diet he would be expected to follow to his own food plan afterwards. Food addiction, he asserted, would not derail him this time.

Options for Treatment

Obesity and Emotional Eating Disorders

Other than twelve-step groups, there are few proven sources of help for the food addict who wants to quit. As we have seen in previous chapters, this is largely due to the challenge of diagnosing the causes of obesity and disordered eating. Is the patient suffering from a hormonal imbalance? An eating disorder? Food addiction? All three? This is the conundrum for any condition that does not have a clear diagnosis: How can you treat something you have not identified correctly? Or, in the case of food addiction, that you have not even considered as existing?

This chapter will cover the treatments that are offered in established clinical venues. The next chapter will address the alternative treatments that are not widely practiced, but that I believe are the most suitable for the food addict.

Typically, medical professionals have resorted to a shotgun approach to obesity and disordered eating in general. Prescribing multiple treatments, clinicians try to cure their patients, hoping that one of their approaches will lead to improvement and that the success of one venture will point to the appropriate diagnosis. Aside from the largely disappointing results obtained with this approach, it boggles the mind to consider how many hundreds of thousands, perhaps millions, of dollars may have been wasted chasing the wrong treatments and getting little success, while the one treatment that shows phenomenal success — abstinence from specific trigger foods — is neglected.

In the medical field, there are three primary approaches to the treatment of obesity and disordered eating in general: surgical, pharmaceutical, and behavioural. Some of these are effective for short-term weight loss, but since none addresses the more complex issue of *addiction,* they are not likely to be effective for a food addict over the long term. If you have attempted one of these treatment approaches and continue to struggle with your weight or your eating, this may indicate that you are a food addict. Most people try many approaches to solve their eating issues. Food addicts often have to try all the traditional options first before they are willing to try my alternative recommendations.

Surgical Treatment

Bariatric surgery is part of the spectrum of surgical procedures devoted to relieving the burden of obesity. Amongst medical professionals, bariatric surgery is often considered the most effective for the morbidly obese. This is often what people want to try first: the effects of rapid weight loss can be quite dramatic and tremendously satisfying. However, if the food that has contributed to the previous weight is not changed, the return of weight is almost inevitable. There are currently four types of surgery available:

1. intestinal bypass;
2. laparoscopic adjustable gastric-band;
3. duodenal switch; and
4. stomach stapling.

For each of these surgeries, the goal is either to obstruct food intake or to limit the absorption of food. The ultimate goal is to force weight loss by making it harder for the body to take in calories.

The intestinal bypass, the oldest form of bariatric surgery, involves a hospital-based surgeon cutting and sealing off a portion of the stomach. This leaves only a small pouch, capable of holding about one ounce of food.

A newer and more popular form of bariatric surgery is the laparo-scopic adjustable gastric-band, or "lap-band," procedure, which also attempts to reduce the size of the stomach. As we saw with Alexander, in this procedure a sterile loop with an expandable inner ring is placed around the patient's stomach and is adjusted to the patient's specifications. At its tightest, it allows for one half cup of food, rather than the six cups a normal stomach will hold. These surgeries are increasingly being per-formed in private, ambulatory "cosmetic" clinics.

A third form of weight-loss surgery is the duodenal switch. This hospital-based operation involves shrinking the stomach along its outer curvature and rerouting a long section of small intestine. The small intes-tine is the site of most of our food absorption, so when this is bypassed, fewer calories are absorbed.

The final type of bariatric surgery is stomach stapling. For this type of surgery, the hospital surgeon uses both a band and staples to reduce the size of the stomach. Today, surgeons often prefer the lap-band because it doesn't require cutting into the stomach, making it a safer alternative. It also allows many procedures to be performed on an outpatient basis, away from the constraints of a tight operating schedule. As it is, wait times for hospital surgeries are typically between three to ten years.

Of patients who have these surgeries, 50 percent report successful weight loss in the first two years, typically losing somewhere between thirty and just over one hundred pounds. Doctors in the United States now perform more than 220,000 bypass surgeries each year, triple the number performed in 2001.[1] Canadian obesity expert Dr. Yoni Freedhoff estimates that in Canada, 6,000 such surgeries were done in 2013 under publicly funded health care.[2]

Physicians tend to advocate for surgery. The benefits are incontestable. The success stories are powerful — patients who have *never* been able to lose weight finally do. Diabetes is cured, high blood pressure normalizes, back pain is relieved, and knee pain decreases. Scooters can be permanently parked. Self-image and confidence increase, depression subsides, relationships improve, and work life becomes more satisfying.[3] Who can argue with these results?

But these good results happen *only if the patient loses weight.* The sad reality is that a significant percentage of patients never lose even five to ten pounds. And for those who do, only about 40 percent are able to successfully maintain their weight loss at the five-year mark.

The key factor that determines success, most surgeons agree, is if the patient *follows the recommended diet and exercise plan.* Otherwise, they tell patients, the weight loss will be short-term. They urge patients to avoid high-caloric drinks and sugary, starchy, and fatty foods. This usually means that patients are expected to change the types of food they've been accustomed to eating in the past.

It bears repeating that surgical treatments only limit the *amount* people can ingest; the *type* of food they eat is regarded as their own responsibility, and the challenge of changing a diet to a healthier one is left to patients to confront on their own. Remember Alexander? This was where he felt the most adrift. Other than a few pamphlets, he received little guidance on what to eat after his surgery. There was no counselling or encouragement to help him with the drastic lifestyle changes that were required to maintain his weight loss.[4]

Given the limited success of these procedures in the long haul, the complications of bariatric surgery are especially ominous. These include everything from difficulty swallowing and indigestion to feeling bloated, nauseous, and constipated. Other medical conditions can follow: nutritional deficiencies, lactose intolerance, gallstones, dumping syndrome, even depression and suicidal ideation. Forty percent of patients develop *new* medical problems after their procedure.[5] Because of these concerns, strict eligibility criteria have been implemented to ensure that procedures are not done haphazardly or for merely cosmetic reasons.[6]

More serious complications can result if the lap-band erodes the sides of the stomach. While surgeons have improved techniques for installing these over the years, at least 30 percent of patients suffer surgical complications and 20 percent of these have required further surgery to deal with these complications. A Belgian study found that nearly 50 percent of patients, like Alexander, had to have their lap-bands removed within twelve years. One to 2 percent of gastric bypass patients have even died during surgery or soon after, and another 5 percent died within a year of the procedure.

Another unexpected complication that has occurred for many bariatric patients is the development of a post-surgery addiction. Fully 6 to 8 percent develop alcoholism or drug dependencies within a year of the procedure. One study has confirmed what we routinely see in clinics: there is a higher risk of alcohol abuse among patients *after* undergoing bariatric surgery. Another study published in *Obesity Surgery* in 2017 claimed up to one third of surgical patients experienced *new onset* alcohol abuse after bariatric surgery.[7]

Dr. Mitchell Roslin, a bariatric surgeon working in New York, explains this phenomenon to ABC News: "A gastric bypass patient has a small pouch [for a stomach], so alcohol goes straight into the intestine and is absorbed rapidly. The higher absorption rate makes alcohol more addictive." One patient reported that before his surgery he could have two drinks, feel sleepy, and go to bed. After the bypass operation, he said, the alcohol would go through his system faster, making him want to drink more.[8]

Despite these real risks, I do not oppose bariatric surgery in every case. I ask only that candidates choose surgery wisely, with a full understanding of the facts about what they can and cannot expect. If they are food addicted in addition to being obese, surgery is, at best, a short-term solution. Unless the compulsion to eat is addressed, food addicts will find countless ways to circumvent the surgical restriction of the stomach: a diet full of sugary foods such as soda or creamy smooth ice cream easily slides past the tight band and will quickly destabilize any momentum created by the initial weight loss.

I am not alone in my concerns. Connie Stapleton is a bariatric and addictions psychologist who is on a similar mission.

Like many of us in the field, Connie is a recovering food addict and alcoholic. She attributes her alcoholism and addiction to pills from the anorexia she developed as a young girl. Family strife, she recalls, led to a focus on food restriction to the point where she lost so much weight she reached 89 pounds. Then her focus on food shifted to drinking and a heavy reliance on codeine pills. Ironically, Connie now claims her addiction to these other substances saved her life.

Connie is still not clear if her initial anorexia was an actual eating disorder or instead a feature of her addiction to food. Sometimes she thinks she just has a severe case of obsessive compulsive disorder that has focused on food and eating behaviours. Obsession is certainly part of her experience, whether it be eating or drinking or abuse of codeine.

Now in recovery from drugs and alcohol, Connie still feels haunted by an obsession with sugar and other trigger foods. To maintain an equilibrium, she has developed her own program of avoiding particular trigger foods and relies on cognitive therapy as well as exercise. She knows the value of group support and has for many years followed a peer support community program.

Fourteen years ago, Connie got a letter in the mail from a local bariatric surgeon who was looking to franchise his work. He needed a counsellor who had experience in marketing as well as addiction. As the psychologist on the surgery team, Connie would do the counselling and group therapy sessions with prospective clients. She took the job, intrigued that the obesity surgeon wanted a counsellor with her skills in addiction. This job seemed tailor-made for her.

It did not take long for Connie to realize that the typical one-hour sessions scheduled for pre-op and post-op clients did not meet the needs of most clients. She started to make YouTube videos to accommodate all the post-op patients. She wrote copious posts on social media to address the multitude of questions her patients had: What could they eat after surgery? Why were they stalling on their weight loss? What should they do in social settings when offered foods they couldn't eat? How do they deal with food cravings and their emotions? Were they allowed to drink?

She wrote a book, *Weight Loss Surgery Does Not Treat Food Addiction*. Her latest project is a Facebook LiveChat, *Food Addiction: Fair and Firm*, which she launched a few years ago. Here she hosts a chat to an audience of hundreds of attendees. In an effort to respond to the overwhelming demands of bariatric clients, Connie has found her niche.

Connie is loath to leave people like Alexander in the lurch. She wants prospective clients to know that obesity is a chronic condition, and that if people do not understand the nature of obesity and especially food addiction, weight regain after bariatric surgery is inevitable. To avoid the disappointment, she wants people considering bariatric surgery to know it is not the solution, but only the first in a long series of changes clients must undergo to maintain their long-term weight loss.

Connie acknowledges ruefully that most patients, even those who self-identify as food addicts, do not want to hear about quitting sugar or their favourite foods. Gingerly, she teaches them cognitive therapy techniques and behaviour modification while still encouraging food abstinence. She also knows she does not have the resources to "clean out the emotional closet" of each client. There is sometimes loneliness, anger, even rage behind the obsession with food, a terrible shame around eating, and behind that often an even greater shame of sexual abuse or childhood neglect. Removing the comfort of addictive foods can be like opening Pandora's box.

Nevertheless, Connie is determined to see that bariatric clinics be mandated to introduce psychological interventions like hers. She is doing what she can for her clients, face to face, on social media, in her books, and even with letters she writes to reluctant clinicians in the bariatric field. Many are hostile to her message of food addiction and the psychic trauma behind food and eating. But in her mind, bariatric surgery without these considerations is unethical.

Pharmaceuticals

At one time, pharmaceuticals were the Holy Grail when it came to disordered eating. Each year, drug companies announced new medications designed to aid in weight loss. Although it is difficult to determine exactly what portion of the annual $40-billion American diet industry is attributable to pills, ABC News estimates that figure to be $18 billion, or almost half.[9, 10] There are approximately twenty-nine thousand varieties of appetite suppressants alone. However, while the general consensus is that a "silver bullet" medication would be a blockbuster, so far medications have produced disappointing results. According to clinician Robert Lustig, whose 2012 book, *Fat Chance: Beating the Odds against Sugar, Processed Food, Obesity and Disease*, is considered a manifesto in the field, many pharmaceutical firms have closed their obesity research programs, searching for greener pastures.

Traditionally, appetite suppressants have been the mainstay of weight-loss medications. These include amphetamines such as methylphenidate (Ritalin) and dextroamphetamine (Dexedrine). While these stimulants curb appetite, they have other serious consequences. The increase in the body's metabolism that occurs with these drugs contributes to weight loss but also creates insomnia, anxiety, and, in some cases, paranoia. Ephedrine was taken off the market for this reason, although I suspect the other reason is that it is the key ingredient used to make the street drug crystal meth. Several very popular appetite suppressants — flenfluramine (Ponerax), dexfenfluramine (Redux), and fenfluramine/phentermine — were all withdrawn in 1997 for their potentially fatal cardiac side effects.

Although the FDA has cautioned against using Vyvanse as a weight loss aid, it is a favoured agent for the treatment of obesity. The stated purpose of this bestselling drug is to help manage the impulse control of a person suffering ADHD and, most recently, binge eating disorder. While its aim is not to suppress appetite, I believe this is the reason why the drug has been successful at producing weight loss. Provided a patient keeps taking the drug, they can lose up to ten pounds. As soon as the patient stops taking the drug, however, often due to the side effects of insomnia and anxiety, appetite and weight gain return.

Another drug, Orlistat (Xenical), prevents the absorption of fats in the small intestine. By inhibiting the pancreatic enzyme lipase, the intestinal tract is rendered unable to metabolize fat, which instead passes through into the stool, thus avoiding weight gain. However, it also causes unpleasant consequences like fecal soiling and incontinence. For many people, losing perhaps only twenty pounds or so doesn't seem worth these socially limiting side effects.

The pharmaceutical industry placed much hope on hormone-altering medications. Focus was placed on Leptin, an injectable version of the satiety hormone leptin. After an injection, the patient quickly feels satisfied with no urge to overeat. But Leptin also diminishes the sensual, rewarding experience of eating, one of the pleasures of life for most of us.

While Leptin has been helpful for people who have biological leptin *insufficiency* due to an endocrine disturbance, it has not helped the many obese and overweight people who end up suffering leptin *resistance*. Injectable Leptin is of no use to a person who already has abnormally high levels of leptin due to his abundant fat cells. Recall that fat cells produce leptin to indicate that no more food is required. Pharmaceutical companies are currently searching for a drug to counteract leptin resistance by making us more leptin *sensitive,* but so far attempts have met with little success. At this time, the only way to restore leptin sensitivity is by constructing a food plan that looks remarkably similar to the food plans I recommend for food addicts.

Another injectable hormone is pramlintide (Symlin). This drug mimics amylin, the hormone released by the pancreas to aid in the feeling of satiety. Many diabetics are deficient in this hormone. At present, the drug is only approved for diabetics. However, experiments are underway to determine if this may one day be useful as another treatment for obesity.

Approved by the FDA in 2014 for obesity and Type 2 diabetes, Liraglutide (Saxenda, Victoza) is yet another injectable that acts like a hormone. This drug mimics GLP-1 (a Glucagon-like peptide), which serves to suppress appetite, but side effects include dangerous hypoglycemia, pancreatitis, and even thyroid cancer. One wonders if these risks, plus the cost of $1,000 per month for the medication, warrant the promised 12-percent weight loss of body fat.

Metformin (Glucophage) is another drug used to treat diabetics. Its function is to moderate insulin resistance, a phenomenon believed to be the major cause of fat accumulation. Insulin is required to transport glucose to the brain. The excess sugar that is not used for energy is transported to the fat cells for storage. A person who is insulin resistant has abnormally high levels of insulin, which have the net effect of increasing hunger and weight gain. Metformin improves the insulin resistance typical of Type 2 diabetes. Since people who suffer from obesity also suffer from a type of pre-diabetic insulin resistance state, this drug has been explored as another option to prevent weight gain as well as to curb hunger pains.

Thyroid medication is also being used to treat obesity. Patients who suffer from low thyroid levels have a sluggish metabolism. This means that their body does not burn calories at the normal rate, which results in weight gain as well as feelings of mental and physical lethargy. Giving Eltroxin to people who have low thyroid levels will make them feel energetic and alert. Giving the drug as a metabolism booster to people with normal thyroid levels may lead to the desired weight loss, but can trigger a host of side effects such as agitation, insomnia, diarrhea, tremors, and even the "buggy eye" swelling typical of someone suffering from Graves' disease (a type of hyperthyroidism that creates an abundance of thyroid hormone). Moreover, if the hormone is introduced to the body through medication, the body's own need to make it will be suppressed (since there is more than enough in the medication) — any interruption in the drug, however, will result in the person developing hypothyroidism (thyroid deficiency) when they were not before.

A whole other category of medications is called selective serotonin reuptake inhibitors. SSRIs are antidepressants, and they work on the principle that increased serotonin from the drug will address the deficit that is apparent in both those who are depressed and those who are obese. Depressed people often overeat to balance their unnaturally low serotonin levels. People who are obese also have unnaturally low levels of serotonin. Giving the drug to correct the insufficiency may take away the need to self-medicate with food.

Drugs in this group include sertraline (Zoloft), an antidepressant that is also prescribed for obsessive-compulsive disorder, anxiety disorders, and bulimia. Another is topiramate (Topamax), a mood stabilizer that is used to treat seizures or prevent migraine headaches.[11] To the delight of the pharmaceutical industry, Topamax was found serendipitously to aid in weight loss. For this reason, it is now prescribed on an "off-label" basis, but it has the unpleasant side effect of making people feel listless and cognitively foggy, earning the nickname "Dopemax" from many users.

Drugs used to block cravings have also been explored. Naltrexone (Depade; ReVia) is a powerful opiate blocker commonly prescribed to decrease cravings for alcohol or to dampen the powerful gratification experienced by addicts of opioid-based medications and street drugs. But it also seems to reduce cravings for food, especially sugar. A similar drug, sibutramine (Meridia), was hailed as a great success until it was taken off the market due to an increased risk of heart attacks and strokes associated with its use. Rimonabant (Accomplia), which blocks the endocannabinoid system that gives marijuana smokers "the munchies," was another promising anti-craving drug, but it too was pulled from the market due to grave safety concerns.

Contrave is the most recent drug from this category of anti-craving medications. Sporting the combination of Bupropion (antidepressant) and Natrexone (anti-craving drug), it attempts to target both the mood and craving disturbances related to overeating. Its success is lacklustre, with only ten pounds of weight loss after one year.

In 2012, two more diet drugs were approved by the U.S. FDA. Lorcaserin (Belviq) boosts the serotonin levels of the brain, triggering feelings of satiety and satisfaction.[12] The manufacturer promises that people can expect to lose twenty pounds using this drug. Common side effects are headache and nausea, but more serious concerns have been listed in the fine print: Belviq can cause tumours in animals and heart-valve defects in humans. Recall that fenfluramine, a similar serotonin booster successfully used for weight loss and appetite suppression in the 1990s, was taken off the market in 1997 due to the same heart-valve concerns.[13] It's difficult to understand why we are seeing such a drug again, especially when these drugs also have addictive potential and can cause LSD-like reactions.

Qsymia is another drug recently approved by the FDA. It is an appetite suppressant that looks like a refurbished phentermine with Topiramate added into the mix. Concerns have been raised about this new combo drug, with claims being made that it causes everything from birth defects and suicidal thoughts to depression, poor concentration, high blood pressure, constipation, memory loss, and insomnia. These drugs carry such serious risks that the FDA initially hesitated approving them, but by May 2013 the FDA had placed both drugs under the Controlled Substances Act.

Behavioural Therapy

"I did therapy for years and years," says one food addict. "My therapist and I talked about everything — my marriage, my kids, my job — while I sat there weighing at least fifty pounds more than I should have. The day I left therapy, he turned to me and said, 'You know, you really should do something about your weight.' How ironic that the one issue that really *was* killing me was totally ignored."

Therapy typically addresses the emotional issues that are believed to trigger eating problems. It takes many forms: individual or group counselling, classic psychoanalysis, aversion therapy, psychodrama, cognitive behavioural therapy (CBT), and incentive motivation. More programs will proliferate once clinicians become familiar with the new binge eating disorder criteria found in the *DSM-5*. It is also likely that, as food addiction becomes more widely acknowledged, more behavioral clinicians will be drawn to serve this population of addicts.

CBT is perhaps the most popular psychotherapeutic treatment. It is used to treat both people with eating disorders and the obese, alongside recommended dietary changes and increased exercise protocol.

Techniques include goal-setting, self-monitoring, stimulus control, and behavioural "contracting" with a therapist or other person to whom one is accountable. We saw this approach with Ruthann, in Chapter 10, who contracted with her therapist to eat a specified amount each day, sometimes under her therapist's watchful eye.

Other components of CBT might include teaching overeaters how to identify thoughts and feelings that lead to overeating and how to prevent or deal with setbacks. Karen, whom we met in Chapter 6, learned how to recognize her trigger foods and how to circumvent her binges by incorporating distractions, affirmations, and mindful eating practices.

Contingency management (CM)[14] is another form of behavioural therapy specific to addiction. This type of therapy has been shown to be particularity effective for cocaine abuse. The program involves "rewarding" good behaviour. To treat disordered eating, a person is rewarded whenever she exhibits signs of healthy eating. Researchers at the University of Connecticut Health Center have studied CM as an option for treating obesity and suggest that it appears to be quite effective, especially among children. They recommend providing rewards not just for weight loss, but also for activities such as keeping a food diary, exercising, cooking healthy meals, and counting calories.

Food plans to guide problem eaters are usually offered within these programs. They include a variety of foods, from healthy greens to small portions of sugary desserts. The philosophy behind CM is that, by addressing disruptive emotions and correcting poor eating habits, the dynamic of disordered eating will be altered, increasing the likelihood that eating *all* foods will be possible. Restricting trigger foods is discouraged, since advocates of CM believe doing so increases the chance that patients will relapse back into their former pathological eating behaviours of counting calories and bingeing.

Cognitive Therapy with a Twist:
Using Reason to Combat the Food Addiction "Gremlin"
Rational Recovery (RR) is an interesting variation on the prevalent cognitive therapy model. CBT is favoured by medical clinicians and has been used for many psychiatric conditions, spanning depression, anxiety, PTSD,

personality disorders, and more. Rational Recovery represents cognitive tools suited to addiction counsellors and their clients.

Unlike Cognitive Behavioural Therapy, which supports a moderate eating plan as its goal, RR counsellors use this model for food addiction to support an abstinence food plan. They encourage clients to use their reason, willpower, and cognitive tools to maintain their abstinence over the long term. Willpower is used not to moderate the intake of tasty foods but to deal with the cravings so that the food addict will not succumb to temptation and end in a food binge.

Rational Recovery is a community-based support network that prides itself on providing an alternative "rational" approach to the belief-based protocol of twelve-step programs. Recognizing the need to avoid the trigger drug (or alcohol or food), the ultimate therapeutic goal is to use rational techniques that support sobriety. There is no need to acknowledge a higher power as the twelve-step program does; rather, one strives to embolden their own will. Indeed, the mainstay book of this movement, written by RR founder Jack Trimpey, is called *The Small Book*, to counter *The Big Book* of AA.

Once achieved, it is possible for an individual to remain sober *without* a long-term support network and a need to believe in anyone other than oneself. Indeed, a person does not even need to label himself an addict once he has made the decision to stop using the substance.

Once the addict understands the true dynamics of addiction and has developed cognitive techniques to command the inner demon (called the Addictive Voice Recognition Technique [AVRT]), she can choose to stop using, even seeing the addiction as a thing of the past. There is no need to be concerned about relapse. Now freed of the obsession and armed with the knowledge that it would be "stupid" to use again, the fully recovered addict can give her attention to other aspects of life. No more meetings, no more addictive behaviour, no higher power other than your own frontal cortex, your own ability to choose rationally.

Florence, a young woman in her early thirties, describes her experience using this model. She is certain she has been a food addict from the start. She ate sugar as a child and when she started to gain excess weight as a teenager, she started to diet. The deprivation inevitably led to bingeing, which led to physical consequences: "I got terrible acne and migraines that required heavy duty pain drugs," she says in our Zoom online interview last fall. "I was so depressed I wanted to die."

She was thrilled to discover William Dufty's *Sugar Blues*. An avid reader, Florence had been trying to understand why she couldn't stop bingeing on foods that clearly caused her distress. When she stopped eating sugar, she discovered to her delight that her acne cleared up, her weight dropped, her spirits improved. Despite all the good it did for her, she nevertheless struggled with her cravings for sugar. This struggle felt like it was coming from an "inner gremlin" that wanted sugar all the time. It raged daily and simply didn't feel like an eating disorder. The diagnosis suggested in *Sugar Blues* felt right. It was a turning point for her to realize that she might be a sugar addict.

She joined a twelve-step program for two years and was pleased with her results but was troubled by the relentless focus on food. She was expected to count her food quantities, weighing and measuring for life. She still felt trapped in the focus of food and eating and longed to put her attention elsewhere. "I didn't want to be thinking about food all the time."

Ever resourceful, she continued to seek alternative measures. She organized the Sugar Summit of 2017 and met Jack Trimpey of RR. She read Kathryn Hanson's book *Brain over Binge*. Here was an approach that acknowledged her food addiction and gave her a rational approach that would enable her to deal with that inner addictive voice (the AVRT) she called her "inner gremlin" for good. She was intrigued by the RR concept that she could split herself between her better judgement and the addict within.

Once she recognized the potential for distancing herself from her inner gremlin, Florence could rationalize herself into sobriety. She would choose from the strength of her higher self, what Trimpey would call the frontal rational approach, to browbeat her addictive voice into submission and sobriety. "Why would I give in to you?" she would ask the addictive voice and dismiss its persistent false promises.

Using the cognitive approach that she adapted from RR, she eventually developed her own model, which she calls the *Sugar Freedom Formula*. Florence knows now that she can not eat sugar, ever, and with her formula, she insists that she has recovered from her addictive food behaviours. She is not *recovering*, but *is recovered*. There is no need for further meetings or support from a higher power. It is a decision she made, and she is now able to devote her attention to other issues. Food binges are part of her history but no longer part of her day-to-day life.

She admits she occasionally still gets cravings or thoughts to eat, and douses these effectively with the techniques from her cognitive tools. Armed with her success, she is now a sugar freedom coach, urging those who do not want the twelve-step support or focus on eating behaviours to try her *Sugar Freedom Formula* as an alternative.

Societal Changes: Turning the Focus Outward

Robert Lustig, Professor of Pediatrics in the Division of Endocrinology at University of California and Director of the Weight Assessment for Teen and Child Health, has worked for years to develop a strategy for treating childhood obesity. Alongside his proposed meal plan, which includes reducing calorie-dense, nutrient-poor foods in favour of low-carb fibre-rich foods, he also calls for behavioural changes in his patients. He requests that they go to stress-reduction classes and participate in moderate to vigorous exercise for at least fifty minutes a day. These activities can help correct the hormonal disarray that sugar has caused in many susceptible individuals.

Although it is not his intention to address food addiction directly, I believe that Lustig's recommendation to reduce sugar and high-density carbs has contributed to the success of his program. Whether the patient is a "carboholic" or a food addict, either is compelled by sugar to overeat to the point of destruction. When sugar in the diet is withdrawn, recovery from cravings and illness occurs.

Increasingly, Lustig is interested in challenging society at large. In an effort to *prevent* rather than only treat obesity, he recommends societal polices that support:

- infants to be breast fed for at least six months (thus avoiding dubious sugar-saturated formulas);
- schools to provide sixty minutes of moderate to vigorous exercise daily;

- clinicians to teach parents and children the importance of healthy diets, stress management, and strong relationships; and
- schools to restrict unhealthy food choices.

Thanks to advocates like Lustig, there is now heightened awareness of the sugar industry's infiltration into health care and government. In his successful book *Fat Chance* and his viral YouTube video "Sugar: The Bitter Truth," Lustig confronts the sugar and food industry head on. Calling out the food industry means we are no longer focusing on the individual. We are no longer blaming the victim. Instead, we are looking at the perpetrators and demanding change.

While the therapeutic approaches highlighted in this chapter are helpful for many, they rarely provide cures for end-stage food addicts unless an abstinence food plan is encouraged. They are certainly worth trying. Karen, who is not a food addict, found peace with her bulimia as long as she continued using the CBT tools her therapist recommended. She is proud that she is able to eat all her favourite foods without bingeing.

Alternatively, Florence is able to live a life free from sugar obsession, provided that she maintains abstinence from sugar. She applies her tools so that she does not slip and "take the first bite" back to misery and loss of control.

Similarly, Ruthann readily admits it is only when her food addiction is addressed head on that her therapeutic advances are not sabotaged by her food cravings. Because she does not safeguard this first step of sobriety, despite ongoing intense group and one-on-one support, she continues to struggle.

For the end-stage food addict, no amount of willpower, affirmations, planning, fear, or bribery can withstand the powerful addictive impulses. These are sparked by the sugars and starches found in the food plans of well-meaning therapists. It is only when those trigger foods are *restricted* that the food addict has any success with these tools. Stopping the food is the first essential step toward recovery.

CHAPTER THIRTEEN

FIRST THINGS FIRST: STOPPING THE FOOD

"You can't just stop eating!" This is the familiar refrain I hear every time I take questions from audiences at my public talks on food addiction. "Of course not," I say, "but you can stop eating sugar, flour, and processed foods, and you can stop drinking soda."

For anyone who has stepped over the line between overeating and addiction, the first step in recovery is to eliminate the drug that is causing the addiction. Just as with other addictions, whether they involve alcohol, drugs, or gambling, treating food addictions requires that the addictive agents — the foods that serve as triggers — be identified and terminated. Of course, abstinence from all food is impossible, and food addicts often say that whenever they eat they are taking the "tiger out of the cage."

The first task is to identify which foods spark the addictive pathways. Sugar leads the list. In a number of surveys of late-stage food addicts, approximately 90 percent identified sugar as the key food they had to eliminate in order to recover from their cravings and compulsive eating. Most of the food-related twelve-step fellowships that can demonstrate long-term success recommend that members completely eliminate sugar.

The next item on the list is usually flour. While many understand that sugar is toxic, people are less likely to identify flour, especially in its "healthy" disguises, such as whole-wheat pasta or multi-grain breads, as a danger. It seems to be the refined nature of flour itself that is the problem. Stripped of their fibrous husks, wheat, rye, and oats are all rapidly metabolized, delivering a high load of sugar and so spurring the same addictive cravings as sweet foods.[1]

Some clinicians and health specialists and researchers pinpoint wheat as being a particular problem. They claim that the gluten in wheat promotes an opiate-like response in the brain. Small wonder that many people find savoury food items like breads, bagels, and pretzels just as addictive as their sugary fare.[2]

Foods that are high in fat are also suspect. Scientists have found that high-fat foods, just like sugary foods, create disturbances in the dopamine and endorphin receptors of rat brains. It is not clear just how addictive fat is, since so many of the fatty foods that are believed to be addictive contain the tasty combination of fat *and* carbohydrates. I believe this to be a particularly potent addictive cocktail.[3]

Some scientists believe that it is the highly processed oils in many fatty foods that are addictive. Many food addicts restrict their fat content as a result, but this is not an essential requirement for food sobriety. Indeed, the human body and brain require nutritional fat for optimal functioning. I do not think that all fats should be eliminated; it is better to be selective about which fats to eliminate. Particularly unhealthy ones, such as trans fats and some saturated fats, should be avoided.

Another substance that recovered food addicts avoid is salt. In the rooms of Overeaters Anonymous and other twelve-step food-related fellowships, you will often hear members talk about their addiction to sweets, breads, pastas, and also to salty and crunchy "savoury" foods. Experimental animal research indicates that salt alters the same reward pathway as sugar and fat.

There is very little *clinical* research available today to support our claims that food is addictive. Most studies demonstrating that sugar, fat, and salt are addictive are still in the experimental stage. Research on rats and mice, however, as well as SPECT scans of humans (which visualize active brain pathways), suggest that food is addictive. I expect that more and more research will be conducted on humans once the medical field formally acknowledges food addiction.

The medical research community may be slow to react, but very sophisticated research is being done by the food industry to identify the "bliss point" in each food it engineers. This is the perfect mix of salt, sugar, and fat that will make the processed food not just tasty but irresistible. In his 2013 bestseller *Salt, Sugar, Fat: How the Food Giants Hooked Us*, Michael Moss wrote that the big food companies' "relentless drive to achieve the greatest allure for the lowest possible cost has drawn them, inexorably, to these three ingredients time and time again. When we hear that the industry is keen to create "heavy users" who will drive sales, we think they really mean "food addicts." As Moss writes, "If sugar is the methamphetamine of processed food ingredients, with its high-speed, blunt assault on our brains, then fat is the opiate, a smooth operator whose effects are less obvious but no less powerful."

Food scientists spend a great deal of time creating what author David Kessler, in his 2009 book *The End of Overeating: Taking Control of the Insatiable North American Appetite,* calls "hyper-palatable eating." Kessler, a pediatrician and former commissioner of the U.S. Food and Drug Administration, talks about how the food industry deliberately manipulates this triumvirate of sugar, fat, and salt, adding them to all its foods so that consumers will be compelled to buy products. He makes the comparison between the addictive products of the "Golden Triangle"— Thailand, Myanmar (Burma), and Laos — where most opiates are produced, and the three addictive substances that the food industry engineers into its products.

Unfortunately, this information is not widely accessible to the public. It is neither generated through the usual research protocols nor published in academic literature. But it's not necessary to find the neurobiological or epidemiological evidence showing the impact of these blissful concoctions. The proof is found not in statistical measures but in sales, in the success of blockbuster food items like Cheez Whiz, Cocoa Puffs, and Dr. Pepper soda.

Another ingredient recovered food addicts recommend avoiding is caffeine. The medical profession has long recognized caffeine as an addictive drug. Doctors regularly encourage patients to moderate their caffeine intake to prevent insomnia, anxiety, stomach complaints, or palpitations. Although you would have to drink about eighty cups of coffee in one day in order to receive a fatal dose of caffeine, drinking more than the recommended two cups a day will cause symptoms of caffeine intoxication and withdrawal, which includes headaches, decreased alertness, irritability, and fatigue.

Some food addicts claim that caffeine can lower an individual's resistance to trigger foods, leading to relapses. They also suggest avoiding the many foods that contain caffeine, such as tea, soda, chocolate, and even some medications. One tablet of an anti-inflammatory medication can have as much caffeine as a cup of tea.

Many food addicts find that they need to stop taking artificial sweeteners, too. This includes all of them, from aspartame, saccharin, sorbitol, and sucralose, to stevia. And, yes, it even includes natural sugar substitutes like honey. Addicts have found that replacing sugar with other sweeteners does not change their weight or their cravings for sweets in the slightest. They just end up eating more, under the mistaken belief that sweeteners do not affect insulin, glucose levels, or weight. We know this is not true. A recent study has shown that artificial sweeteners *do* alter insulin levels, thus stimulating weight gain.[4]

In the early days of Overeaters Anonymous (OA), many members used diet drinks and the blue-and-pink packets of Equal and Sweet'n'Low, but they found they started to binge on the artificially sweetened foods. For food addicts, anything that goes in the mouth — from cough drops to sugar-free mints, from candy and chewing gum to chewable antacid or Pepto-Bismol tablets — can become a problem.

As one OA member, who no longer uses sugar or any other sweetener, recalled: "I was using two dozen packets of artificial sweetener a day until a massage therapist, of all people, said the only way to cure a sweet tooth was by giving up anything too sweet. I was amazed when I ate unsweetened oatmeal and even yogurt and they tasted wonderful."

There is now science that says most laboratory animals and some humans can be addicted to artificial sweeteners. In tests with cocaine-addicted mice, the mice preferred sweetness over cocaine. Judging by my colleague Phil Werdell's clinical experience, this science explains many of his clients' problems with soda. Since 1986, he reports he has worked with over four thousand late-stage food addicts and hundreds of self-assessed food addicts who could not stop bingeing with the help of therapy or twelve-step programs — until they removed artificial sweeteners and caffeine completely from their diets.

The most common problem was diet soda. Food addicts considered these drinks safe when they were dieting because they contained no calories. Even when addicts practiced abstinence from sugar as a part of a food addiction recovery group, they kept drinking their diet sodas and they kept relapsing, returning to sugar. With this particular subset of late-stage food addicts, eliminating diet sodas was a part of the strategy to achieve stable food abstinence and food addiction recovery.

The food addicts I know found their way back to recovery only when they eliminated these replacement treats. "I only became willing to give up sugar-free mints after I was reduced to lying on the floor of a public bathroom because I had such abdominal pain from the sorbitol they put in those things," says one addict. "I was eating, not chewing, packs and packs of them every day, telling myself that they were okay because they were 'sugar-free.'" Given the power of its addictive qualities, it is not surprising to learn that cocaine-addicted rats were found to prefer artificially sweetened water to cocaine almost 100 percent of the time.

Phil's Story Continued

Twenty-six years ago and a hundred pounds heavier, I ... sought out recovered food addicts. It was suggested that I eliminate completely all my binge foods. I wrote them down: there were seventy-six. With some difficulty I abstained from them for a few days and noticed that I didn't binge. One of my binge foods was sugar-based soda. I abstained from sugared soda by drinking artificially sweetened soda and from coffee by switching to decaffeinated coffee.

About twelve years later, I started having trouble with diet sodas and decaf coffee. I was drinking more of them, sometimes even when I had made a commitment not to do so. Then, one day, I went into a grocery store and picked up a six pack of regular Coke, not diet. A recovering food addict I was with noticed and I took it back. Soon after, I started drinking whole pots of decaf coffee at every meal. I was unwilling to stop until I got some help from a recovered food addict.

The detox was the most difficult I have had with any food, possibly because I was so clean from other addictive foods. But I am now completely convinced that I crossed over the line into physical craving for artificial sweeteners and the small amount of caffeine in decaffeinated coffee.

While Phil's story illustrates the power that specific ingredients can have, food addicts have also told me that the *amount* of food they eat can be as triggering as the food itself. Many are not able to estimate appropriate portions since their drive to eat overpowers any true hunger and satiety signals. They experience the phenomenon of "false starvation," whereby they misinterpret their craving for the buzz of food as hunger.

How do you know when you are full? One person may only need two pieces of chicken to be full, whereas the food addict may find that two *halves* of a chicken still isn't enough. These addicts need the discipline of using a food scale or a set of measuring cups and spoons to measure portions of food. That way, whether they feel hungry or full, they eat a predetermined amount of food each meal. It is medically necessary, but, sadly, they often face scorn and criticism when they do this in public.

Still, despite the inconvenience of carrying around these utensils, the benefits far outweigh the problems associated with a potential for relapse if the addict is left to her faulty judgement. It is, after all, possible to binge on so-called "healthy foods," whether carrots, celery, or even water. As one addict explained, "Weighing and measuring gives me freedom." Enjoying appropriate portions, she said, "takes away the fear and the guilt about food.... It quiets the chatter and the back and forth about whether my food is too much or too little. It's worth it."

Having someone prepare and serve the food may be especially useful for the food addict who has a history of anorexia.

Detox

Once addictive foods have been identified, the next step is to abstain from these foods. What does abstinence mean exactly?

Since sugar is universally identified as a major trigger, detox usually means removing any *added sugar* from a diet. But for some people, this may not be enough to get free from food cravings. In fact, many find that most processed foods contain too much sugar. Some find recovery only when they eat foods in which sugar is listed as the fifth (or lower) largest ingredient in the food and that the items do not include multiple forms of "hidden" sugar. This means going to the effort of reading labels and learning the different names that sugar can go by: high fructose corn syrup, dextrose, fructose, evaporated cane juice, barley malt, etc.[5]

Eating healthy, unprocessed foods is a start, although it may still not be enough. Not all foods — even those considered healthy — are created alike. How quickly a food breaks down into sugar can be just as important as whether it contains added or hidden sugars. The glycemic index measures how quickly food is broken down into sugar, so the higher the glycemic rating, the more sugar is present to make that food addictive.[6]

Even fruit can be problematic. Many people find they need to abstain from fruits that contain high fructose loads, like mangoes, bananas, and cherries. This is especially true if the fibre has been removed. Juices are an excellent example of drinks that are as toxic as soda. I recommend that these be eliminated. Corn, peas, potatoes, and yams are vegetables that are also high on the glycemic index and can cause problems for some people.

I encourage people to eat foods with a low glycemic load, such as cauliflower or broccoli. The goal is to maintain an even blood sugar level, rather than to have levels that spike up and down. This is usually accomplished through a nutritionally balanced food plan with plenty of green and brown vegetables, proteins, and fats. If you still have cravings, you should try to identify the food that is still driving the addictive cycle.

It may come as a surprise to you that some people find they also have to eliminate dairy products, even healthier items like skim milk or yogurt. Do you ever wonder why some people really love their yogurt and cottage cheese? These contain natural sweeteners in the form of lactose and casein, which our stomach breaks down into casomorphin, an opioid peptide that some late-stage food addicts find addictive.

Identifying particular trigger foods beyond the usual culprits of sugar and high glycemic foods such as flour and fruit can be a process of trial and error. A successful food plan must be tailored to each person's unique history of food abuse and the severity of her food addiction. A good rule of thumb for food addicts new to recovery is to abstain from all trigger foods until cravings are removed.[7]

The temptation to reintroduce these foods back into a food plan will emerge at some point. We live in a world populated by people who cannot fathom a diet of no flour or sugar. Food addicts will eventually be tempted to become less rigid in their eating. Personally, I have found the peer pressure of maintaining a diet free from sugar and carbohydrates to be far more daunting than the simple act of not eating them.

Reintroducing trigger foods at any point, even after years of food sobriety, can drive an addict back into addictive eating. A simple "cheat" here and there, even the smallest nibble from someone else's dessert plate, can reintroduce cravings that will undermine months, even years, of good behaviour. It is usually in the stage two Maintenance phase that most Weight Watchers dieters fall off the wagon. Most people are surprised by how quickly they return to overeating and how rapidly they regain their weight.

Food addicts will only find recovery once they have identified all the trigger foods unique to themselves and have eliminated them from their diet. Only then can they hope for freedom from their addiction. But before reaching that place of food serenity, there is a no man's land of withdrawal and increased cravings that all addicts must endure. Post-acute withdrawal syndrome (PAWS) will try even the most resolute amongst us.

Withdrawal

Withdrawal occurs once a person stops eating any addictive food. Abstaining from trigger foods will cause a level of discomfort that often drives addicts back to eating. Symptoms might include headaches, anxiety and irritability, feelings of being too hot or too cold, depression, sleepiness, or difficulty in sleeping at all. It really depends on the addictive food. If the bag of jellybeans provided an excited rush, lethargy will follow. If the ice cream provided a numbed feeling of lassitude, then anxiety and irritability will often follow once the effect wears off.

Feelings of deprivation, obsessions about food, and anxiety arising from unresolved trauma that was being "medicated" by the addictive foods may appear like specters that linger, worsening before they get better. The food addict in withdrawal is like a Tibetan "hungry ghost" — an insatiable creature with a tiny throat and a bloated stomach.[8]

During this period, addicts report that it is as if the addiction has a mind of its own, and that it senses the end is near. Says one food addict, "It's weird — [it's] like all my foods know they are going away and they make one last, desperate attempt to get back in my brain." Another recovered food addict describes "Having this disease … it's as if I have two people in one body."

It may seem that life without one's comfort foods is simply not worth living. Even problematic eating is seen as better than feeling bereft to the point of suicidal thoughts. But others might find the symptoms so common that they are not even recognizable as withdrawals. I am convinced that many people mistakenly attribute their ongoing depression and anxiety or bipolar symptoms to an inherent genetic disorder that requires medication; I think their mood disorders may actually be the manifestation of the addictive cycle derived from the foods they are eating.

Cravings are the hardest to manage. These translate into the insidious thoughts that whisper to the addict: "Have just one more as a final treat;" "I will start again tomorrow;" "I need this in order to work, sleep, take care of my kids;" "I can control myself this time...." These addictive impulses can weaken even the most determined person.

The good news is that detoxification isn't a long process. A complete "cold turkey" detox from all trigger foods (as opposed to a gradual abstinence) only lasts between one week and four weeks. If strong cravings last longer than a month, it might be that the food addict is still eating an unrecognized trigger food — something is still feeding the addiction, thus prolonging the withdrawal process. A person who stops eating sugar may not have eliminated *all* forms of sugar (as mentioned earlier, these can range from artificial sweeteners, like Sucralose or dextrose, to honey, concentrated fruit juices, or the hidden sugars in ketchup, mustard, and sauces). They may need to abstain from starchy vegetables like potatoes or yams, which rapidly metabolize into sugar during digestion. Persistent cravings are often a sign that some food is still sparking the addictive pathway.

Cheating by having a bite here or a spoonful there is also an excellent way to suffer withdrawal in perpetuity. Withdrawal will not end if the substance is constantly being reintroduced into the brain reward pathway. This is perhaps one reason why a gradual detox that does not eliminate the trigger completely is actually more difficult than a cold turkey approach.

An excellent resource on how to detox and manage withdrawal symptoms is Dr. Nicole Avena's 2013 book *Why Diets Fail (Because You're Addicted to Sugar)*. This book not only presents hard science on sugar addiction, but also gives an eight-step plan on how to go sugar-free. It is an excellent primer to help the reader determine which foods to eat and which to avoid, along with how to navigate the obstacles that can occur in the first four difficult weeks of post-acute withdrawal from sugar addiction.

Successful detox is not usually done alone. As with most addictions, withdrawal from food addiction is best endured with the support of others. Willpower often crumbles in the face of overpowering urges. Unfortunately, such support is rarely available.[9]

Cold Turkey Detox

One organization that provides help for food addicts during detoxification is ACORN Food Dependency Recovery Services.[10] A five-day residential workshop, ACORN's Primary Intensive program is an alternative to in-patient treatment for those who do not need hospitalization or direct medical supervision. ACORN, which operates in cities across North America, usually holds its workshops in private homes with up to twelve participants. The workshop includes education about the disease of food addiction, opportunities to identify and express difficult feelings, and an introduction to the type of spiritual work offered by twelve-step food-related fellowships.

However, the main purpose of the Primary Intensive program is to offer a five-day period of abstinence. From the first day, attendees learn how to eat abstinently, taking all of their meals together. Although a variety of therapeutic interventions are offered throughout the week, those dealing with issues of physical abstinence always take priority. It is necessary to attend to such issues first, because a person still caught in the loop of addictive thinking is unable to reap the benefits of any therapy or education that might otherwise be very powerful. The addictive thinking will dominate and obstruct the insight and judgement required to make use of these interventions.

Participants learn to commit themselves to a food plan that eliminates the major addictive foods: sugar, flour, excess fat, and caffeine. Once each participant has identified his own particular binge foods, he removes those, too, from his diet. Such foods can include anything from sugar-free chewing gum to chicken skin to popcorn. If an attendee does not already have a food plan that has worked for her, she is given a healthy eating outline, such as the one devised by author and food addict Kay Sheppard or by Theresa Wright.

Wright is a nutritionist in the U.S. with decades-long expertise in food addiction. Her specialty is to devise a menu plan that isolates and removes trigger foods while ensuring that the medical and nutritional needs of the attendee are met. She is adamant that one menu cannot fit all needs: male, female, pregnant, and post-bariatric clients may all require individualized tweaks to their food plans for long-term success.[11]

ACORN'S meal and therapeutic program is based on the now-defunct food addiction residential treatment program that was offered at the Glenbeigh Psychiatric Hospital in the 1970s. ACORN's success is resonant with Glenbeigh's, which found that up to 90 percent of their patients succeeded at staying abstinent if they followed the recommended program's *Healthy Eating Plan.*[12]

Similar results were found with the participants in Renascent's food addiction program. Renascent is Canada's largest residential addictions treatment centre, offering month-long treatment at three sites in the Greater Toronto Area in Ontario. From 2015 to 2017, it conducted a year-and-a-half long pilot project, admitting almost eighty residents into its food addiction program. Food addiction clients lived side by side with other clients who were there to recover from alcoholism, cocaine, or opiate addiction. Preliminary research from this program showed the majority of clients who complied with *all* the recommendations, beginning with the abstinent food plan, were successful. Those who continued to use a food buddy to hold themselves accountable to their food plan and who attended aftercare group supports are still abstinent one to two years after treatment. As is said in recovery circles: "It works if you work it."

A Renascent Food Addiction Grad: Wendy's Story

Wendy started hiding food when she was ten years old. Even at that age, she was embarrassed to admit the amount of food she could eat. She was teased about being the biggest girl in her class. The taunts made her cringe and want to eat more. By the time she was a teenager, she had discovered how to diet. Like everyone else who cut down their favourite foods, she found that she would gain even more weight back once she resumed eating her forbidden foods.

Wendy was baffled why she would eat to the point of feeling nauseous and bloated. After each binge, she promised herself that she would stop eating "tomorrow" but found that "food would be the first thing on my mind again upon awakening."

By the time Wendy, who is five-foot-four, heard about the Renascent food addiction pilot program, she weighed 293 pounds and was desperate. She was even willing to try residential treatment. She was so anxious, she told me, that she ate non-stop in the car all the way to the treatment centre. She stood outside the front door of Renascent's downtown residence, across the street from the Art Gallery of Ontario, still holding her bag of binge food. It was as if she could not let it go. After a long moment, she rang the bell.

Her stay was successful. Away from her triggers and responsibilities, she relished the month that allowed her to focus only on herself. At last, she could detox from the sugar and flour, absorbing the support of the counsellors and her fellow patients, without "being left to my own devices." She loved the intensity of classes from morning until night, which kept her from emotions that lurked beneath. She appreciated the extreme measures the centre put into place: whenever a resident left the building, staff searched their bags on return to make sure the clients did not smuggle in "contraband" food. Wendy felt protected from her inner conniving addict. To her delight, she discovered how the women in the treatment centre who struggled with alcoholism and drug addiction were just like her. "I felt welcome, like I belong there too." They were all just addicts.

Wendy left Renascent armed with an abstinent food program and recovery tools to prevent relapse. Abstinence now, she tells me, "is not eating any sugar, flour, or grains, and eating only three meals a day with no snacks in between." Wendy knows that following the food plan is not enough, that she is not just on another diet. She has to maintain daily safeguards around her eating regimen as she returns to her previous life. She attends an online biweekly support group of Renascent alumni. She goes to OA meetings, conventions, and workshops. She calls a sponsor every day and uses all the relapse prevention tools she has been given. Fourteen months later, Wendy is still abstinent and she has lost over 100 pounds.

Wendy lists the miracles she has achieved in this last year, which she is certain she would not have achieved if she had not walked through the doors of the residential program. "I can do things I've not been able to do in years," she tells me, teary with appreciation. "I enjoy my meals more than ever before, and all of my cravings for junk are gone … and I don't have to crawl up the stairs in my house anymore. I don't have to nap each day just to get through … I can do up my seatbelt!" She is amazed that she is off her medications.

Another bonus is that Wendy now loves to shop. No more plus size stores. She is no longer afraid that she will be the largest person in the room whenever she goes out. Most of all, she is thrilled that she is able to help others. "I feel great," she says, beaming. "I'm finally living my life again."

Like ACORN, Renascent provides a "cold turkey" refined carbohydrate detox for the first five days. Within a week, the client is introduced to a meal plan that is both nutritious and sustainable for the rest of that person's life. There is no staging of specific plans (from a strict low caloric amount to a permissible one) that is typical of many other programs that focus on weight loss. In fact, most clients on arrival are amazed and pleased at how much food they are expected to eat. While the detox period feels grueling to some, no one feels hungry or deprived of food.

And difficult those first five days of detox can be. Lesley, another grad from the program, claims that she could not have made it without living in a residence where she was surrounded by others who were there to help her. Whenever she had detoxed in the past, she would get sick, have headaches, and find she could not focus on anything. She would feel jittery and inevitably go back to eating sugary food. "If I had been at home without the support of the other ladies in the house I would have quit trying. Knowing from others' experience that these feelings would pass kept me going."

The Renascent program includes medical supervision and dietary surveillance for the many clients who are post-bariatric or who have diabetes and high blood pressure. It has become routine to expect changes in a client's medications once she is eating well again. Mental health also improves. It is remarkable how quickly clients achieve a level of physical and mental health within only three or four weeks of healthy eating. For many, insulin, antidepressants, and stimulant medication are no longer necessary once the addiction has been addressed.

On top of eliminating the consumption of sugar and flour, the Renascent program also removes grains such as rice and oatmeal from the diet. Clients are taught to weigh and measure meal portions. Thus the centre presents a program that spans the triggers of most end-stage food addicts, with the possibility of fine-tuning the meal plan once the person has left the program. In some cases, with the guidance of a food buddy, a client may be able to reintroduce caffeine or sweetener, or make slight changes to food portions if too much weight is lost.

In addition to the food plan, Renascent also integrates participants into its larger addiction program. Food addiction clients live side by side with other clients who are dealing with substances such as alcohol or cocaine. They attend many of the same classes, troop to the same evening twelve-step groups in the community, and plan to attend the continuing care program to ensure familiarity with relapse prevention techniques for after they leave the residence.

The underbelly of much substance use, including food, is trauma. The alcoholic or cocaine addict often relies on food to detox from their drug of choice. Counsellors encourage this when they suggest that the alcoholic eat candy whenever a craving arises. What can the food addict rely on? Food is often the *last drug* a person has to let go of, and when that is removed, there is no buffering the underlying trauma. Trauma-informed Renascent staff were regularly called up to teach basic grounding techniques for the food addict panicked about their newfound emotions.

Teri, another Renascent grad, says her struggle with eating always includes regulating the strong emotions tied into her food behaviour: "I was battling severe trauma that I had experienced in my past." She explains that she was "desperately trying to remedy the internal strug-gle between weighing and measuring my food and my past unhealthy eating behaviours and restrictions. I was angry that another person or place was trying to control my every move, including when and how much I could eat. Being a bit of a control freak made this aspect of the program extremely difficult." Counsellors and fellow patients helped her get though these hurdles that she would not have even attempted on her own. Food and trauma are often so intertwined that trying to detox and stay sober in the face of painful emotions is daunting. She knew she could not do this alone.

Teri was abstinent for five months after leaving the program. However, one day, she sipped wine at a Catholic communion, and the old cravings emerged. Suddenly she was off her pink cloud and was free-falling back into the abyss of her previous bingeing. Just as before, "I was on my couch at home, eating." Before she knew it, "I was dying and yet I could not stop bingeing. I got winded walking, tying my shoes, just moving, period."

Teri wants to return to residential treatment. She says adamantly, "For me, I need to be locked up in order to stop my binge eating." She comes to the centre weekly to attend outpatient classes, hoping to get back the strength she found when she was an inpatient. She feels the support from the centre and the Renascent alumni community is integral to her potential recovery.

A number of food addiction alumni who are still abstinent agree. Uniformly, they say that they are only able to maintain their abstinence one year later by going to OA meetings, following the Renascent food addiction alumni Facebook page, and participating in twelve-step study groups.

This steadfast support worked for Lesley: "Now I smile a lot." She no longer suffers from sleep apnea or needs to take her blood pressure or GERD medications. She isn't depressed. Instead, she's ziplining, tree-top trekking, snowshoeing, kayaking, hiking, and singing in a women's choir. She's back in school, working toward her dream job to become a nurse. She has a life she never imagined possible. "I'd forgotten that life could be this good," she concludes, with a big smile.

Unlike Renascent, which positions itself as treating disordered eating *solely* from an addiction model, most other residential centres that treat food addiction are forced to provide a dual diagnostic approach in order to receive funding. Insurance pays for addiction care or for eating disorder programs — but not both. Hence these centres may use services from within their eating disorder *or* addiction programs to offer a sub-stream of service that caters to the food addict.

Some of the better-known residential American programs that provide similar forms of support are the following:

- A six-day session at Shades of Hope in Buffalo Gap, Texas
- Weekend and seven-day workshops conducted by Kay Sheppard at Kay's Place, Palm Bay, Florida
- The COR food recovery program, offered by The Retreat, Wayzata, Minnesota
- A week-long stay at Rebecca's House, Lake Forest, California
- The Intensive Program for eating disorders and food addiction at Turning Point, Tampa, Florida
- A month-long program at Milestones in Recovery, Cooper City, Florida

What all these programs have in common is that they help an active food addict become sugar free and binge-food free. They teach clients about food addiction and usually introduce a twelve-step program. Treatment programs generally follow the same food plan, though there may be some flexibility in how the initial abstinence is implemented.

Would you rather jump into the cold swimming pool quickly and quit all trigger foods at once — as is typically done in a residential setting — or would you prefer to gradually dip one foot in at a time?

Some food addicts need to disengage from one substance at a time — first sugar, then flour, followed by sweeteners. They require a more flexible approach, especially when it comes to what is sometimes a deal-breaker: the practice of weighing and measuring of food in restaurants or during social occasions. Such an easing-in can be done in the community where it is best to detox in a less drastic way, especially without the counsellors, set meal plans, and support to help the addict through the tortures of sudden withdrawal. The end result is the same: those who follow the detox food plan and maintain the guidelines of no sugar, no flour, no trigger foods, and even the weighing and measuring foods, will likely succeed in staying abstinent. The sooner this goal is achieved, the quicker the cravings and obsession associated with food disappear.

What CAN I Eat?

"If I stop all my addictive foods, whatever will I eat? What kind of diet must I follow?"

This is always the first question I get from people when I speak publicly about the nature of food addiction. People crowd around the podium, acknowledging they are food addicts but puzzled as to what to do next.

I do not recommend a specific diet. There is no temporary solution to the problem of being overweight. There are literally thousands of diets and they are, for the most part, finite programs of caloric restriction. Typically, they have three stages. Stage one involves a reduction of high-fat and high-carb foods; stage two allows for a gradual reintroduction of the problem foods; and stage three involves a restricted but more permissive consumption of most foods — including the trigger foods that can stimulate compulsive eating.

Readers in the addiction field will be familiar with the concept of harm reduction.[13] This concept involves trying to moderate the use of an abused substance rather than insisting on abstinence. There are clinics that provide "clean" heroin to users or teach them how to safely use the heroin they acquire; there are hostels for older alcoholics where they permit moderate drinking and even supply alcohol to those who can't afford it. We claim that this approach is analogous to what is advocated in the typical diet plan. Addicts are taught to moderate their "drug," whether it is alcohol, heroin, or sugar, so that they consume quantities that are not considered dangerous for them. How harmful can a few cookies a day be? The little harm they may cause is minimal in exchange for the benefit of living normally by eating the foods that everyone else can eat.

This reasoning does not allow for the frenetic, compulsive nature of addiction. Although some designers of diets acknowledge that several foods are addictive, none of the diet literature proposes the most successful cure for food addiction. Instead, abstinence is considered a poor alternative to the moderation plan. Some experts even view it as pathological.

I don't share this view. That's why the food plans I endorse replace the notion of moderation with abstinence. Some foods are addictive and need to be avoided. Eating in recovery, therefore, involves more than a change in the choice of foods; it involves a fundamental change in attitude. My choices of food follow this philosophical shift in how I view eating.

I believe that the diets proposed by the low-carb or paleolithic diet communities are fairly sound. They are ideal for food addicts or anyone who would like to follow a healthy diet free of addictive foods. Most of these meal plans encourage a protein-rich, vegetable-based diet that contains a moderate amount of fat for satiety.[14] The goal of these plans is to decrease insulin spikes that drive hunger, cravings, and obesity.

The food scheme proposed in *Why Diets Fail* by Dr. Nicole Avena follows the same principles: discourage *all* processed foods, since these contain the sugar, fat, and salt combinations that drive people to eat in unhealthy and addictive ways. Tony Vassallo's JERF (Just Eat Real Foods) food plan, found in his *Weight Loss Never Tasted So Good,* is another such approach. He advocates a sugarless, flourless food plan with portion control. If you are a food addict, you may need to alter these plans slightly, as some allow for natural sweeteners such as honey or stevia.

Books such as *The Blood Sugar Solution 10-Day Detox Diet*, by Dr. Mark Hyman, who is himself a recovered food addict, can also be helpful. His proposed detox follows the same principles of avoiding sugar, flour, and processed foods, emphasizing instead lean proteins, veggies, nuts, and seeds. He also encourages the adoption of other lifestyle changes to support his food plan, such as stress reduction, exercise, nutritional supplementation, and social connection.

The sample food plan below is built around this principle of abstinence and has been designed with food addicts in mind. It is similar to the Renascent plan. Note that this schema eliminates sugar, flour, and grains and requires weighing and measuring of food portions. Keep in mind that individuals have different needs according to their histories and the stage of their food addiction, and that this plan may need to be tweaked.

Many commercial and twelve-step programs recommend a generic plan, so that members can start from a common template. They have found that these plans have achieved the best long-term success for their members, and suggest that their fellowship follow the guidelines for at least three to six months before attempting to make any significant changes.

A Food Addiction Basic Food Plan

Breakfast	Lunch	Dinner	MA (METABOLIC ADJUSTMENT)
	(4 hrs. after breakfast)	(5–6 hrs. after lunch)	(4–5 hrs. after dinner)
1 protein/ dairy (4 oz)	1 protein (4 oz)	1 protein (4 oz)	protein/dairy (2 oz)
1 fruit (8 oz)	1 cooked vegetable (4 to 8 oz)	1 cooked vegetable (8 oz)	or 1 fruit
nut/seed (1 oz)	1 fresh vegetable (8 oz)	2 fresh vegetable (12–16 oz)	or one fat
	daily oil (1 oz)	daily oil (1 oz)	

These portions are subject to change if a person has had bariatric surgery.

The recommendations in other food addiction plans may differ slightly, but all are based on the premise that sugar and flour are the trigger foods that must be avoided for lasting success. Some of these diets recommend further restrictions, such as avoiding sweeteners or weighing and measuring food intake. One of these plans may be your first crucial step toward a life free of food obsessions and the real possibility of serenity.[15]

Slippery Abstinence

"Slippery," or imperfect, abstinence is better than no abstinence at all. For addicts who have stopped eating sugar and flour but find that their cravings are just too intense to resist, I suggest that they look at their diet more carefully. Cravings and slips are usually an indication that *something in the food plan* is still causing a trigger. Are there any new binge foods and hidden sugars? Dairy can cause relapses for some addicts. Kay Sheppard, author of *Food Addiction: The Body Knows*, explains the first three things to do if you are in relapse:

- check the food,
- check the food, and…
- check the food.

I cannot stress enough that hidden food triggers are the most overlooked reason for relapses, and their presence may indicate that you have not fully detoxified. Registered dietician Theresa Wright, who has helped countless food addicts, finds that many of the clients she deals with have items in their food plan that can cause low-level cravings. She tells relapsers to ask themselves: Which specific food or foods am I overly attached to? Which food(s) am I most unwilling to give up?

Grains can be acceptable for many food addicts. However, at Renascent, we have discovered that over time, even after years of food abstinence, some people find that grains do become triggers for food cravings, and are the cause of the creeping five-to-ten-pound annual weight gain that happens post middle-age. Healthy grains such as wild rice, quinoa, and oatmeal seem to cause difficulty once a woman reaches a certain age, typically around menopause. Perhaps this newly emerged sensitivity to grains illustrates the slow, progressive nature of addiction itself. Even while the food addict eats a clean food program, sensitivity to particular foods increases. Many of our clients have found that their stubborn weight plateau and food cravings dissipated once grains were completely eliminated.

A secondary addiction may also be sparking off the food addiction. Some people are what we call "double and triple winners," which means they have another addiction paralleling their food addiction. Common co-addictive substances are marijuana, alcohol, cocaine, prescription drugs, and diet pills. Process addictions can include co-dependency, sex and love addiction, compulsive exercising, workaholism, compulsive spending, and gambling. These can all spark off each other. After a beer, the drinker craves pretzels; a win at the slot machines calls for a huge dessert. We suggest that "double" food addicts address their dual addictions simultaneously.

Just Say No! Pitfalls to Abstinence

Even with support, the struggle to avoid trigger foods involves a number of obstacles that make it hard to withstand detox and long-term sobriety. It is worth listing these, since they can undermine recovery.

Perhaps the biggest struggle comes from within the medical community itself. Doctors and dietitians schooled in the notion that obesity is caused by a lack of self-control usually balk at the concept of abstinence. They declare that abstinence creates a sense of deprivation and will foster binge behaviours. If a patient has a history of an eating disorder, medical providers are often convinced that restricting particular foods and measuring portions will firmly entrench the eating disorder pathology.[16]

Most medical clinicians prefer to encourage people to eat *all* foods, including sugar, in moderation. Food addicts who present their abstinence treatment plan are often discouraged, *even if their plan is working.* The irony is not apparent to health professionals: Would that same clinician urging moderation of sugar insist that a crack addict learn to smoke crack in controlled amounts? Advise a cigarette smoker to cut down to just three cigarettes a day? It is the rare person who once smoked a pack a day who can gradually reduce their habit to three cigarettes a day without undue emotional strain.

Doctors and dietitians also voice concern about the nutritional soundness of a diet that is abstinent of sugar and flour. There is a prevailing belief that a healthy diet must contain healthy whole grains and flour. Thankfully, most health professionals are reassured when they examine our proposed diet of green and brown vegetables, proteins, and healthy fats. They might be surprised to see that their patients could even be eating *more* calories, since they are no longer engaging in fasts to lose weight.

Health professionals are especially delighted when they see the results of this food plan, which are often nothing short of miraculous. Their patients are transformed from being morbidly obese, with life-threatening conditions such as diabetes, major depression, heart disease, and serious joint problems, to becoming happier people with normal weight and negligible health concerns.

The societal attitude toward diets in general presents another major obstacle. The term *diet* is usually understood to describe a temporary change in eating that is expected to last only until the end goal of weight loss or diabetic control is met. Rigidity is frowned upon; the occasional lapse into sugary, fatty foods is expected, even encouraged. "You have to relax a little" is the advice often offered to those unwilling to step out of their plan for the occasional snack.

Disapproval is greatest when food addicts pull out their scales and measuring devices at local restaurants. "Aren't you taking that too far?" "Are you *still* doing that?" Even food addicts flinch, second-guessing themselves, as they notice the wary glances of others at nearby tables. Yet, for food addicts, these techniques of sobriety guard against their temptation to overeat *or* undereat. A scale could be the difference between momentary discomfort in public and the onset of a relapse that could last for years.

If you are a food addict, the information in this chapter may seem daunting. The list of tempting foods to avoid can be formidable, the spectre of going through detox unnerving. If finding residential support is not possible, how will you manage to soldier through the three weeks of detox and all the hidden traps ahead that may lure you back into a relapse? You may be pleased to know that there are an increasing number of recovery solutions in the community. The next chapter will highlight some of the options most suitable for your circumstances.

CHAPTER FOURTEEN

RECOVERY IN THE COMMUNITY

How Judy Collins Conquered Her Cravings: The Easier, Softer Way

She was a world-famous singer, a beacon of peace and love, the blue-eyed personification of all that the 1960s meant in America. Yet she punished herself with alcohol, drugs and most of all, food. She threw up. She starved herself. She tried every diet ever conceived by man or woman. She gained and lost hundreds of pounds.

She fought depression as a child and even once tried to kill herself by ingesting 150 aspirin tablets. As a result of her erratic eating, her bones suffered and her menses often stopped. As a teenager she showed no signs of overweight, yet she lived to binge on sugar products and junk food — pies, cakes, chocolate-covered cherries, popcorn, homemade treats and soda.

Thirty years of therapy didn't help. While her career as a folk singer soared, her eating and drinking worsened. She kept it all a secret, damaged her health, and threatened her livelihood with addictive behaviors that impacted her voice. Giving up the alcohol and drugs with the help of a twelve-step program gave her a measure of stability, but the eating continued. At that point in her life she says she was "sober but drunk with the food."

Finally, she hit bottom. At the end of a day during which she had stuffed herself with candy bars, doughnuts, cookies, sweet breads and sugared nuts and purged at least five times, she dragged herself to the only place she could think of that might help: another twelve-step program specifically for food.

It was there that Judy Collins, the popular singer and bestselling author of her narrative, found relief. By surrendering to the same principles that had helped her give up alcohol and drugs, she began a journey that included detoxing from all sugars and adopting a weighed and measured food plan focused on fresh, whole foods.

Today, Collins is the author of an autobiography, *Cravings: How I Conquered Food*. In it, she chronicles her travels through various food-related anonymous fellowships, until finally settling into GreySheeters Anonymous (GSA) in 2008. She supports any twelve-step program that helps, but has taken issue with the mother of all food groups, Overeaters Anonymous.

When her book was first published in 2017, Collins told the *Huffington Post* that she fell out of love with OA after their board of directors got vague about food plans. "How can a food recovery program not teach you how to eat?" she asked. The OA principle, called *a dignity of choice*, meant that the food plan could include any number of trigger foods.

Collins called her own ultimate surrender to the highly structured plan endorsed by GSA her "salvation." Her abstinence means no sugar, no flour, weighed and measured food, nothing in between three meals a day. She stays away from processed foods of all kinds, as well as her trigger foods — sugar, grains, flour, corn, and wheat. Rather than feel deprived, Collins tells me in a phone interview, "My meals are glorious. I have a huge life in those meals. It truly is the easier, softer way to live." When I asked her if people criticized her approach as extreme or rigid, she laughed, explaining that she doesn't listen to negative comments anymore, adding that "their criticisms are not on my daily food plan!" Communicating her pleasure in her body size and the freedom she experiences from food obsessions is her service to those who are looking for models of success.

Collins' book is really a fascinating two-for-one: she alternates chapters about her own struggles with food addiction, bulimia, and alcoholism with historical profiles of various diet gurus and weight loss trends, beginning with Lord Byron. Names such as Jean Nidetch, Dr. Max Stillman, Dr. Robert Atkins, and Adelle Davis will be familiar to anyone who has tried to lose weight. What may not be familiar is how each expert came to his or her conclusions about how and what to eat.

By including these various approaches to dieting, Collins has (intentionally or not) underscored the notion that there are various ways to lose weight and keep it off. Thousands swear by Weight Watchers, the *Dr. Atkins Diet Revolution*, eating "paleo" (mostly animal proteins), *The Starch Solution*, the DASH diet, etc. So while, like Collins, many food addicts have found help in the halls of twelve-step fellowships, it would be incorrect and possibly even medically unethical to promote that path as the *only* road to recovery.

There are many viable alternatives to OA, FA, FAA, GSA, et al., and as acceptance of food addiction continues to grow — along with the obesity epidemic — it's a good idea to give each and every option a fair hearing. Food addiction is a complicated disease; treating it requires an open-minded willingness to go beyond a self-righteous "one size fits all" mentality. But one common thread in all these approaches is that of a supportive community, a network of human connections that makes the journey through recovery less solitary. And sometimes, if you can't find a community where you feel you fit in, you have to create your own, as the following stories illustrate.

Man on a Nutritional

I met Tony Vassallo at one of my public talks two years ago. Sitting at the back of the room, a tall, slender man raised his hand when I asked the audience who among them had lost weight — and who had kept it off for at least five years. I expected a flurry of hands at the first question, but I knew most would drop at the second. Tony, however, had lost over 130 pounds and kept it off for eight years.

The people in the room turned to look at him. Abashed, he told the onlookers that he had simply quit junk food. The "man" foods, to be specific, such as nachos, wings, ribs, burgers, and fried chicken. Tony attributes his success to not eating those "kryptonite" foods, ever. When he did, he would invariably binge.

Before he sought help from a commercial weight loss program, Tony had been struggling with his weight for some time. Like so many men in his age group, forty-year-old Tony had been gaining weight incrementally each year. He had already been diagnosed with diabetes and frequently suffered painful flare-ups of gout. He knew that obesity in men is especially worrisome and hard to treat.

Some men are predisposed to metabolic syndrome (the trifecta of high blood pressure, diabetes, and high cholesterol), which can lead to other conditions: sleep apnea, heart disease, and even early onset dementia and cancer. While the National Eating Disorders Association estimates that 10 million American men will suffer from an eating disorder during their lifetime, men who need help often don't get it.

When Tony hit 300 pounds, he had had enough. It wasn't the gout or the sleep apnea or the hypertension that frightened him most. It was that number 300. It was then that Tony joined a local commercial weight loss program and lost 130 pounds in two years.

The leader of this weight loss company was so impressed with Tony's success that he asked him to join the team. Tony was thrilled to be a coach. He had already been looking for more meaningful work and now he could help others while doing what he loved to do most: cook. He coached men how to shop and prepare food and hoped one day to write a cookbook.

While Tony had been losing his weight, he had discovered that he had a real problem with sugar. Each time he had a nibble even of "healthy" sugar (e.g., maple syrup, honey), he wound up bingeing. Although addiction was not yet part of his vocabulary, he was learning its mechanics.

However, the food plan that he was expected to promote in his new job did not reflect his experience. Like most programs, it encouraged a moderate food plan that excluded processed foods laden with sugar and flour in the short term, but added them back later. It stressed an "eat less and exercise hard" approach, with a heavy reliance on self-control and exercise. While this "bust your balls" approach often led to substantial weight loss, the macho approach rarely led to lasting results. Tony was not surprised to see success was short-lived for many of his students.

Four years later, a disillusioned Tony decided to leave the commercial program. He wanted to go out on his own with a food plan that he had faith in. He went back to school to learn nutrition and designed a food plan that was nutritious, free of all trigger foods, encouraged portion control, and suggested well-spaced out meals. He called his plan JERF (Just Eat Real Foods) and wrote the book he had been dreaming about for years, *Weight Loss Never Tasted So Good.*

Tony knew that he had needed a solid support group to help him stay clean from binge foods. He needed help to cope with life issues (break-ups, financial insecurity, even food cravings) *without* relying on food. He realized that he felt safer sharing in a roomful of men, so he decided that he would establish a space mainly for men. Thus was born his company, MODA Nutrition, Inc. (In Italian, the word "moda" means style or fashion.)

Tony is not alone in his need for male support. One of the first men who came out publicly as a food addict was Michael Prager, author of a 2010 memoir titled *Fat Boy, Thin Man.* Prager writes candidly about topping out at 365 pounds and getting treatment for food addiction a number of times before finally finding abstinence and serenity. Today he is a blogger, public speaker, wellness coach, and popular talk show guest.

Tony insists that working with men is different from working with women, who typically outnumber men in most food-related twelve-step groups. Special concepts and tools are required. While women are keen to ask questions and are more inclined to take direction willingly, men are usually stubborn at the outset.

"It starts with ego," Tony explains. He says that men have a difficult time admitting they have a problem — with anything. "Asking for help," he adds, "means we need to swallow our ego, in the same way we hate asking for directions when lost in traffic."

To illustrate his point, Tony describes a typical first meeting with a new client. The man begins by rationalizing why he is obese. The newcomer says he is "big-boned," "husky," and has "bad genes." He adds that he is only seeking help because his wife is worried about him. Men, Tony says, rarely ask a friend who is losing weight how they did it, for that would sound like asking for help. It might take weeks for the newcomer to admit that he overeats.

Anticipating resistance, Tony rarely mentions addiction in the first interview. "First," Tony explains, "the man will dismiss the concept with a shrug and say something such as, 'Addiction? How can you be addicted to *food*?' Then, when it occurs to the client that I am serious, he usually gets testy. His eyes widen, he licks his lips, and promises to renew his gym membership. He'll go jogging every day or do *anything* except stop eating sugar and bread or drinking alcohol. Next the client will shriek, '*What? Are you saying NO more pizza, NO chicken wings, NO sweets, NO beer? What do you want me to eat? Twigs and leaves?*'"

Faced more than once with this tension and defeatism, Tony has learned to rely on his former "fat guy" status to gain credibility and make the client comfortable. After all, Tony admits that he *still* sees himself as a fat guy hiding in a thin man's body. "I position my conversations with clients as if I were trying to knock some sense into Fat Tony's head of several years ago," he says.

Tony prefers to use a baby-steps approach, removing just one trigger food at a time, and takes a better-than-before approach when recommending the JERF plan. Tony is especially wary of prematurely introducing the twelve-step language of surrender, because men are expected to be all-powerful. He explains how uncomfortable the feelings of powerlessness and humility (as Step One promotes) can be for a man who is used to being a prosperous businessman. He knows that spirituality (or personality transformation) is integral to long-term recovery from addiction, but he takes a secular approach. Instead of talking about God or a higher power, he stresses adhering to "Pillars," principles such as surrender, belief, honesty, and personal growth.

Tony likes to punctuate the beginning and end of his weekly gatherings with the MODA mantra: "I care about my health and my wellness. I eat real foods in controlled portions at proper intervals. I am the priority." All the men in the class stand up, as if swearing an allegiance to their health, and shout out the mantra in unison. It is a powerful display of fierce individual spirit captured in a group action. At one recent meeting, several men — defeated yet belligerently defiant just one year ago and now at least 50 pounds lighter — enthusiastically applauded each other. In doing so, they gave the new guy peering in at the door a huge dose of hope and help.

Challenging the Bondage of Numbers

At twenty-nine years old, Sandra Elia was at the darkest point in her life. Her marriage was deteriorating, and she was unable to work. She avoided her friends. She weighed 260 pounds. She hated everyone around her, especially herself.

It would start each morning. Reeking of sweat and food from a binge the night before, Sandra struggled to get up. Her muscles ached as she shuddered at the thought of brushing her teeth, showering, putting on her clothes. It all seemed insurmountable.

Seeing the wrappers and bags on the floor as she shuffled to the bathroom always depressed her. But when evening came, she was back on the couch in a dark living room, stuffing herself until she felt sick. Pizza, pasta, bread, desserts, ice cream. "My life," she said of that time, "could be summed up in three words: desperate, hopeless, decimated."

Sandra tried to get help. Over the years, she had tried going to multiple diet centres. She saw doctors, specialists, and dieticians. Nothing helped. "These attempts," she told me in the living room of the Toronto treatment centre where she works, "gave me false hope. I think they brought me further into my addiction."

Out of the blue one day, Sandra remembered a twelve-step food recovery group she had once attended and thought, "Why not?" At the meeting she saw people of all sizes laughing and talking. She came home that night suffused with the feeling, "I am at home. These are my people." And she did not think of eating.

Sandra started to attend the meetings regularly. She appreciated that the members talked about their struggles with food, and she felt liberated to share her own secrets. Although she still overate, the need for food gradually lessened. She knew that some foods could trigger massive food binges, but she was not ready to give them up right away. Instead, she followed a regimen of eliminating sugar first; then, when she felt brave enough, she cut out other trigger foods such as flour and nuts. It took a year for her to identify and quit all of her "poison" foods.

But Sandra was still obsessed with her weight. The peer group she joined was urging her to reach a goal weight that felt tyrannical and unhealthy. She did not want to feel "the bondage of the numbers." Abruptly, she threw her scale in the trash.

"Gone are the days of eating to appease the scale," she told me. "One day I decided that my weight was none of *my* business." Her task was simply to eat fresh, whole foods, and avoid refined sugar and flour. She would stop looking at the number on the scale. This approach was the pivotal point for her success. Today, the scale is no longer able to tell her she is undisciplined, lazy, and ugly. Those hateful thoughts just made her want to eat.

Regardless of her weight, Sandra now seeks a more positive view of herself. She finds that her "affirmative approach is energizing," and has enabled her to funnel her energy into more constructive ventures. She left her "boring" job at a prestigious consulting firm and now works in the field of food addiction. I met her two years ago when she interviewed me for a radio series on obesity and food addiction.

Today Sandra is co-chair of Obesity Canada (formerly known as the Toronto Chapter of the Canadian Obesity Network.) She is one of the first trained and certified food addiction counsellors of the International Food Addiction Counsellor Training program (INFACT) and plans to be one of its future trainers. When the Renascent program put a call out for a food addiction counsellor, I knew Sandra was the perfect match. She has the experience of food addiction recovery that she can model to clients.

Sandra has a strong vision for the future. She wants to build supports to help food addicts detox slowly in the community, much as she had to do herself. Not everyone can get into a residential detox program for food. Since the community supports for food addiction are limited, Sandra is determined to fill that void.

Sandra wants to present a secular alternative for those unwilling to go "into the rooms" of a twelve-step fellowship. She has conceptualized a three-pillar model that captures the foundation of the twelve-step platform in a more contemporary way: elimination of trigger foods, group and one-to-one support, and spirituality and mindfulness. To realize her goals, she is currently working with four outpatient groups at a local weight management and diabetes clinic. She also has a private practice in food addiction, offering an eight-week outpatient program, weekend and five-day retreats, and one-on-one coaching.

Sandra is sharing her experience and hope with others. She has redirected her old self-destructive energy into food recovery instead. Where before she struggled to get off the couch to brush her hair and shuddered when looking at the scale, now she is a fireball of energy and activity. She beams with the energy of a food addict in recovery and is a shining star in Canada for food recovery and sobriety.

A Nutritional Approach: Your Personal Food Plan

Theresa Wright is a registered nutritionist who has been working with food addicts since the 1970s. It all started quite by accident. Nutritionists and dieticians are *not* trained in the field of food addiction; instead, they are trained with the understanding that all foods, even addictive foods such as sugar and flour, are safe if consumed in moderation. A nutritionist, like Wright, who stands outside this paradigm, has risked the wrath of her colleagues — for many years. She has felt the silent treatment during coffee breaks at meetings and has not been invited to attend key conferences. Because of the traditional animosity of dietitians toward the food addiction model, Theresa Wright is perhaps the sole nutritionist in the U.S. who has decades of clinical experience in food addiction.

Although Theresa is not a food addict herself, her background in social psychology helped her to understand the terrifying clutches of addiction. She has also worked in tandem with notable counsellors in food addiction, like Phil Werdell. Theresa became known as sympathetic to the food addiction cause and was even asked to write the manual for OA's *Dignity of Choice*. This document helps members of OA to find an abstinence plan that works best for them.

Given the complexity of food addiction, Theresa is more than a nutritionist. Certainly, her first concern when working with a food addict is to design a food plan: She asks each client, "how would it feel if you stopped eating this food, for two weeks?" If the client shrugs and agrees to stop, Theresa knows that food is unlikely a trigger food. But in our interview she tells me, "I had a patient once get on her knees, begging to not be asked to stop her pizzas.... So, I knew they had to go." She smiled a deceptively cherub-like smile.

Most clients find out what she already knows: that they must get completely sugar, flour, and wheat free. They might even have to stop sweeteners, especially NutraSweet or sugar alcohols like xylitol and mannitol. She will gingerly allow a client six packets of Splenda a day with the aim to see if any food compulsivity returns.

Her 2017 book, *Your Personal Plan Guide*, is a composite of her experience designing food plans. Theresa attempts to address many of the individual nuances that make each plan unique: for example, an individual of short stature might only require 1,000 calories while a pregnant woman may require as many as 3,000 calories. She estimates that people usually range between 1,800 to 2,000 calories. She has also designed a formula to help her clients balance their protein, carb, and fat requirements.

Armed with a unique food plan, Theresa then teaches clients how to shop, prepare, and cook. People often have to start from scratch, learning how to read labels, how to determine what foods are healthy — for example, to distinguish the difference between various yogurts — and to unlearn their fear of fat. She also instructs clients to use scales to encourage portion control. She intuitively knows that for the addict, it is impossible to determine how much is enough. Clients need to learn how to "recalibrate their eyeballs."

Theresa also knows that some people use food to numb the intense emotions that may surface once the food is "quiet," no longer distracting them from their inner turmoil. When this happens, she refers clients to psychologists, trauma therapists, and the twelve-step program. A client may need help with an abusive spouse, or a highly critical boss, or PTSD from early adverse childhood experiences. Sometimes these emotional tumults must be dealt with before long-term sobriety can truly take hold.

Training the Food Addiction Counsellor in the Community

Since *Food Junkies* was published in 2014, a plethora of counsellors and food plans have populated the Internet promising to treat food addiction. I am concerned that, while the popularity of these ventures indicates a public awakening to the phenomenon of food addiction, their solutions are often misguided, and, ultimately, damaging and demoralizing to the food addict.

Unless they have had training in the addiction field, many therapists do not understand the mechanics of obsession and cravings and the necessity of trigger-food abstinence. Instead, they focus on the goal of weight loss or on strengthening willpower. It took a pioneering spirit in Iceland to envision a standardized training program that could teach this essential information to professionals working with disordered eating.

Esther Helga Guðmundsdóttir is a fiery, dynamic woman with an infectious laugh who speaks quickly and with emphasis, a woman of action. From her home in Iceland, she once taught opera singing and even gave lessons to Jónsi Birgisson, the famous voice of Iceland rock band Sigur Rós. Yet for years Esther was secretly miserable with the ravages of her own food addiction.

She was forty-eight years old when she finally experienced the moment of relief that changed her life. Through the trial of several different twelve-step groups, she finally found a food plan that placated the extreme nature of *her* food addiction. She could no longer eat any sugar, flour, or grains, and she needed to weigh her food portions. She had to pull out her scale at restaurants, family dinners, even under the disapproving eye of her friends who scoffed at her rigour. Within this structure, she has been able to happily maintain a weight loss of 150 pounds for more than fifteen years.

Three years into her recovery, Esther felt ready to share her story with others. In 2006, she started a private practice for food addicts offering private sessions, seminars, and group therapy. Located in Reykjavik, Iceland's capital city, MFM Matarfíknarmiðstöðin (MFM Food Addiction Centre) is an out-patient recovery program that has treated more than two thousand food addicts since it opened.

In her work, she discovered that many clients had already tried to treat their food addiction but failed because the treatment did not understand the dynamics of craving and food obsession. A student of Phil Werdell, who began training professionals in the 1970s with his five-day outpatient intensives, Esther saw the need to take his vision further. Her program, the International School for Food Addiction Counselling and Treatment (INFACT), is designed for any professional (physician, nurse, dietitian, therapist, or counsellor) to sub-specialize in food addiction. INFACT opened its doors in 2017 and has already produced fifteen counsellors who now share a common understanding of the disease and treatment of food addiction. I am hopeful that this training program will contribute toward a universal understanding of the dynamics of and recovery from food addiction. Another community, this time of professionals in the field of food addiction, is taking shape.

The Way of the Future? Bright Line Eating, Multi-Media Food Addiction Treatment

Dr. Susan Peirce Thompson begins her story with two marshmallows given to her when she was four. She quickly figured out how to get more by standing on a chair to reach the cupboard where they were stored. She calls this memory the beginning of her descent into full-blown food addiction — "hiding, sneaking, and stealing food." The disease continued, leading her to try multiple food regimens, bulimia, and even drugs such as crystal meth, which curbed her appetite. Finally, Susan found the abstinence that worked for her in a twelve-step program that involved a very structured way of eating, eliminating sugar, flour, and all of her trigger foods.

Like many who try twelve-step programs, Susan eventually became disenchanted with the structure. "I was confronting a common paradox of the twelve-step food community," she says. "If a program is relaxed enough to accommodate a busy life, acknowledging that people have kids and other priorities, the less likely it is to work for any given attendee." In other words, the fewer demands the program had, the less it seemed to work. She reflected that "the programs that seem to work really well for long-term weight loss tend to be rigid, even fanatical, in their approaches." But people often leave these groups saying they are too cultish or infused with a religious fervour that turns them off.

Susan wanted to create an alternative that could fill the gap between the twelve-step programs that promoted an addiction and recovery model that she knew worked and the multiple diet programs that did not. Adapting the principles of what she had learned in her twelve-step program, she created a plan to achieve her ideal body weight and be free of the obsession to eat incessantly.

Today, Susan teaches brain and cognitive sciences at the University of Rochester (NY) and is an expert in the psychology of eating. In 2017 she published her book, *Bright Line Eating*, the blueprint of the eating program that worked for her. Through this book, she is able to bring a program to people who had the very same struggles that she did.

She named her program "bright lines," after the term in law to describe a clear and unambiguous guideline intended to ensure consistent results. She notes that "the principles that I evolved into *Bright Line Eating* were first introduced to me at a twelve-step meeting for food addiction." These guidelines include the popular OA and FA "suggestions" of "no sugar, no flour, weigh and measure." She adds a fourth bright line that reflects a slogan still advocated by some twelve-step food groups: "three meals a day with nothing in between."

In her book, Susan is excruciatingly candid about her eating history, her bulimia, her binges, and her difficulties with losing weight. She also explains the biochemistry, physiology, and neuroscience of food addiction in a way that is enormously helpful to the layperson trying to get a grip on this seemingly innocuous thing called food that can hijack even a highly educated brain. "When I started," she says in an online interview with me, "I just wanted to write a book.... I wanted to get the information out there" about the science of food addiction." Susan was concerned that this information was simply not available to the public.

Susan especially wanted to provide a *flexible* plan in which clients could choose to follow only the aspects of the program they needed. Not everyone needs extreme measures. She designed an "eating susceptibility

RECOVERY IN THE COMMUNITY · 205

scale" that reflects the continuum of addiction: those who are on the lower end of the scale do not require the same abstinence or efforts that those on the other end require, such as residential care or twelve-step programs. Not everyone needs the rigid food choices and portions that she knew she needed for herself. Her program could also help the many people who only need some guidance toward weight loss and might otherwise be turned away by the tougher regimens needed for the more extreme food-obsessed clients.

Broadening the base to serve those with mild addictions (those who score between one and six on the DSM-5's eleven-point scale) means the focus for many clients can be just *weight loss* rather than relieving the relentless obsession with food. *Bright Line Eating* puts a great deal of emphasis on weight. Susan's coaching practice, book, blogs, and the entire social media community she has so successfully built are founded on a *diet*, and on learning how to become "happy, thin, and free." This is in contrast to AA's goal to be "happy, joyous, and free." Susan's book is sprinkled with before-and-after photographs and testimonials from the formerly fat who have gone through the two-week boot camp and the follow-up help designed to help them achieve and maintain their goal weight.

It is too soon to know whether all those pounds will stay lost. If there is one thing a real food addict knows, it's that you are never, ever cured. To paraphrase a popular sentiment from *Alcoholics Anonymous*, "An addict is like a man who has lost his leg. He will never grow a new one." My approach, in contrast, is to focus on the addiction primarily and expect that the excess poundage will disappear eventually. The weight is but a symptom of the disease of food addiction.

Through the multimedia aspect of the Bright Line platform, Thompson has gained great success in the last few years. Her programs exist in various cities in the U.S. and beyond. She claims to have helped thousands to lose weight — thousands who would otherwise not have succeeded in traditional diet programs or managed to sit past the first few meetings of a twelve-step food program. With these numbers, she also hopes to provide data to help clinicians validate that the addiction paradigm really does work for weight loss.

This is not a moot point. A major disadvantage for those who uphold twelve-step programs is their inability to study the success of their members. Anonymity is sacrosanct and embedded in the traditions that define how every twelve-step program is run. Without people recording their names, weights, or personal stories, data cannot be gathered or tabulated. Without data, it is impossible to determine a program's success.

For example, in 2017 the Overeaters Anonymous World Service Office conducted a survey that gathered demographic information from its members as well as recovery rates. According to the OA website, the survey showed that since coming into OA, 73 percent of members had lost weight, and 54 percent of them report that they are currently maintaining a healthy weight. These numbers are impressive, but the methodology used for the survey was hardly scientific: seventy-nine group secretaries were asked to distribute surveys randomly and recipients then went online to record their responses.

We need more experts like Thompson to conduct research in an effort to deal with the naysayers who continue to dismiss the devastating impact of food addiction on individuals, families, and society as a whole. Unlike many twelve-step programs, her secular version allows her to rigorously question food addicts and follow their recovery so that she can study the success of food addiction treatment.

To her credit, Thompson's candour and honesty about her own struggles with food provide powerful proof that food addiction is a chronic, incurable disease. One may be relieved of its horrors, but never entirely cured. On her popular YouTube vlog she tells her followers that she has binged at least twice since founding Bright Line Eating.

One break came on U.S. Election Night 2016, and another more recently at Thanksgiving 2017 after a painful experience with a close friend left her with a lot of emotional pain that she wanted to anesthetize. During that second relapse, Thompson shares that "unmanageability" crept into her life and she "picked up the food" (including sugar and flour) for six days.

What's beneficial from the tell-all approach in her vlog (her "most popular" and "most helpful entry yet," she says) is hearing what Thompson did to get back on track. To use a popular twelve-step phrase, she went "back to basics." Her recovery came full circle, which meant she returned to using the tools that gave her relief from food in the first place and long before *Bright Line Eating* — calling a twelve-step old-timer to ask for help, making phone calls to abstinent friends, committing to her weighed and measured food plan every day. As an addict at the extreme high end of the spectrum, she had to turn her attention from weight to the *addiction itself* if she did not want to regain her weight.

"It's important to me to be a role model for being honest and vulnerable," Thompson says in our interview, adding that her own experience with relapse taught her that she needed to slow down, not travel as much, and keep her focus on her recovery. "Being on the road is really hard... I've learned how profoundly our environment matters."

By combining the old wisdom contained in the twelve steps of recovery with multi- and social-media communication, Thompson has hit on a winning formula. She is able to reach out to a multinational community. She, and others like her, can build connections to a broad community — the essential antidote to addiction.

CHAPTER FIFTEEN

SWITCHING ADDICTIONS

Just 'cause you got the monkey off your back doesn't mean the circus has left town.

— GEORGE CARLIN

"My disease morphed. I stopped drinking and gained twenty-five pounds."

"I quit smoking and started eating like a house on fire."

"After I was able to quit bingeing on food, I maxed out all my credit cards. I just couldn't stop shopping."

"I put down sugar, but now I drink two or three pots of coffee every day. I've become a caffeine junkie."

We often hear these laments from addicts who have been successful in giving up their primary addiction. It is as if addiction is a multi-headed hydra: if one head doesn't bite you, another one will; chop off one head and two more grow back.

"My husband quit smoking," one woman wrote in my online addiction forum, "and now I think he has replaced cigarettes with food. I try to make sure that he is eating a healthy diet. He has a good breakfast and I pack his lunch with nutritious foods. He doesn't always eat everything I give him, but he is eating normally.

"The problem starts after supper," she continued. "He will usually leave a little on his plate, but whether he eats it all or leaves some, he always claims he is full. Within thirty minutes, sometimes less, he is looking for something to eat and will continue [doing] that until bedtime. He used to get up every thirty or forty minutes to go out for a smoke; now he gets up looking for food. It is always bad food.… I am so happy he quit [smoking], but I think he is still addicted. How can I help him?"

This woman is right. Her husband *is* trading his nicotine dependency for another addictive substance. He is using food as if it were a drug to replace his nicotine cravings. The very fact that it works indicates the success of this technique. But the long-term consequences are high. The major concern with using food as a smoking substitute is, of course, weight gain.

The latest estimate is that people who quit smoking will gain approximately ten to twelve pounds. While some of this is because nicotine suppresses hunger (thus the ex-smoker initially feels more hunger and needs to eat more often), much of the weight gain is due to compulsive overeating. Smoking also boosts the metabolism, so even if an ex-smoker quits and doesn't eat more, she may add pounds unless she also ramps up her physical exercise. There is another factor, too. Weight gain also occurs because the bacterial flora in the gut changes from strains that are less efficient at digesting food, such as Proteobacteria and Bacteroidetes, to more efficient strains such as Firmicutes and Actinobacteria phyla. Excess carbs are thus more readily converted to fat. Packing on these pounds can often drive a smoker back to smoking again.

The Power of Substitution: Sugar to Quit Crystal Meth?

Harvey Parra is a forty-two-year-old Mexican American. He is five feet, eleven inches tall and currently weighs 215 pounds. "That is muscle," he tells me over the phone. "I used to be 305 pounds and that was not muscle!" Since I can't see him, I ask him to describe himself. He pauses to think, then declares that he is a laid-back man who typically wears jeans, a simple coat, and tennis shoes. He chuckles that he likes to hug people and play pranks. He is, he says, a people person, well suited to his life as a real estate broker. He loves spiritual music and is a devoted Christian who attends his church at least twice a week.

We conduct a phone interview since Harvey lives in San Diego, three time zones away from me. Several years ago, Harvey had contacted me, telling me how he had quit sugar and changed his life. Many people have contacted me through my *addictionsunplugged.com* website, but Harvey stood out in my memory. His story illustrates how food can be a very seductive substitute for drugs — and even more daunting to quit. My mouth dropped when I heard how he halted his crystal meth use by substituting sugar for it. As an addiction physician, I know that crystal meth is one of the most devastating addictions to combat. "Oh yes," he gravely assured me, "food is a much worse addiction than crystal meth."

Harvey's drug use started in his childhood. He was in and out of hospital due to a bowel condition that required surgery, and he was given morphine as a little boy on a regular basis. "I was a drug addict by the time I was a toddler," he tells me ruefully. "I came to love drugs and how they made me feel." By the time he was in high school, he had accumulated addictions to alcohol, cocaine, and crystal meth. In his midtwenties, he finally sought residential treatment for his hard-core addictions and was successful in getting off the drugs. He stopped alcohol, cocaine, and crystal meth cold turkey. But he ate instead. And ate, and ate. "That's how I quit drugs," he explained, "I used food as my substitute."

Alarmed about his resulting weight gain, Harvey attempted to change his diet. He scoured the Internet and discovered the Atkins program. To his delight, he lost one third of his weight by diligently following that food plan, losing one hundred pounds in the space of two years. "Life was going well," he confided to me over the phone, "except that I was still secretly obsessed with drugs. I was dry." He sighed. *Dry* is a term that addicts often use for the "white-knuckling" feeling that a person who is still hankering for his drug experiences while actively trying to hold back his urges. Usually, it is just a matter of time before the addict gives in again.

Eventually, the inevitable happened: seven years later, after an unhappy divorce, Harvey relapsed. He started to use crystal meth, cocaine, *and* food. In a panic, he struggled to control all three addictions, but it was another eight years before he regained his sobriety. Throughout, he had fits and starts of trying to stop drugs (three months clean, only to start again) and trying to get back on the Atkins diet so that he would not regain his weight. Mystified, he could not understand why anything he did only worked for three months. And he was getting tired of counsellors and friends telling him not to worry about his eating as long as the drug use stopped. He knew that more was needed, but he could not determine what.

Then the penny dropped. In December 2010, after stopping his drug use one more time, he decided to focus his efforts on changing his food choices. He hunted for a solution to his eating problem online: Was there a way he could tweak his Atkins program? He stumbled upon online communities of low-carb dieters and read that many of their programs encouraged the novice to start a new food plan by cutting out sugar, flour, and grains, at least for the first few months. He decided to try this more drastic approach, what he called "Atkins on steroids," reckoning that in the past, while he had cut down his carbs, he had still included modest amounts of bread and other grains. This time, he kept his carb content to the first stage of the Atkins program — which allows twenty to thirty grams of carbs a day. Typically, a person following Atkins can shift to higher levels of carbs after a few months, but he did not budge from the first stage.

"It was hard, Dr. Vera," he admitted. "I had to call upon my personal relationship with Christ, get a one-on-one talk with him, be still, listen to his support, his advice, his encouraging words." He credits his spiritual relationship with giving him the necessary support to get through the withdrawal from both his drugs *and* his food.

The first few months were tough going, he conceded, and it was the *food* more than the drugs that beckoned to him. "I discovered that whenever I stopped using drugs," he said, "the itch, the beast, that wanted me to use crystal meth, would come back after three months, but the beast in me that wanted to eat sugar would be back in three days." It was a relentless itch, a hunger, a void that demanded to be filled. Using his spiritual tools as well as online videos and support blogs (especially the well-known blogs of Jimmy Moore and Kent Altena), he got through those first months without relapsing to drugs or food.

Harvey realized that the major difference between his previous, temporary success at achieving sobriety and his current success was that now he was no longer eating *any* sugar and grains. He refused to reintroduce these, even moderately, at the three-month mark as per the Atkins protocol. To his surprise, he learned that not only did his sugar cravings subside, so did his residual longing for his drugs. It dawned on him that in his past sobriety attempts he must have been inadvertently feeding the addiction to sugar, which in turn "kept the meth and cocaine buzz alive."

This insight was pivotal to his success at remaining sober and resisting *all* his addictions. Before this, as an evangelical Christian, he had always interpreted his struggles with addiction as a kind of spiritual warfare, wrestling with the obstinate, diabolical part within himself that wanted to keep using. Now, he understood that his addiction was physical, not spiritual; there was something biochemical that kept triggering and keeping alive the addictive impulse. Once that was quelled, the addictive impulse would subside. This was not the devil — this was sugar and flour and grains (basically, the simple carbs that metabolized to sugar within minutes).

Since then, Harvey has still had thoughts of using, but he is able to manage these. He gets them mostly when he is hungry or stressed, and estimates that these cravings now feel like a four out of ten in terms of strength, rather than the ten out of ten he experienced in the past.

Harvey admits that he has slipped a few times in the last two years, but each time he has been able to stop before any of his addictions have had a chance to take over. Once, after a breakup with his girlfriend, he confesses that he drove straight to a McDonald's and promptly ordered a soda and burgers. As he wolfed the food down, he could feel the same guilt overwhelming him that he had had with drug relapses of the past. But this time, he knew what he had to do — stop the food.

I ask him what kind of supports he relies on to help him in the face of the multiple temptations that bombard him daily. He is silent and then discloses that he does feel lonely. "Friends and family want to be supportive, one hundred percent," he acknowledges quickly, "but they [have] addictions themselves." I could almost feel him shaking his head. "People," he said bemusedly, "have no idea how addicted they are, they have not been off it [junk food] for long enough … they have no idea." In fact, he sees himself as the light, the example; sometimes he is even the guilt-inspiring reminder that they are not eating healthily. "They want to see but they don't want to."

Harvey foresees that one day there will be more sugar-free rehab programs that will treat addicts who are tempted to switch their addiction to food. "This is why, Dr. Vera," he confides, "I wanted to do this interview. And you can use my real name. This *is* important." Harvey wants to be in the vanguard of a life-saving revolution.

Mark the Gambling Man

It all began innocently enough. Late one Sunday evening, twenty-six-year-old Mark and his girlfriend finished a Thanksgiving family dinner and, looking to end the night with a flourish, they decided to go to the local casino. It was his first time. Mark looked around the room, taking in the slot machines, the whirling roulette wheels, tables filled with trays of food and spilt beer, cigarette smoke permeating the air. Unbeknownst to him, Mark was at the start of an eleven-year love affair with "big money dragon."

Sundays went from regular nights out at the cost of $200 a night, to weekend getaways at full-scale casino vacations over major holidays like Thanksgiving, New Year's, and even Christmas.

Mark isn't sure exactly when his newfound entertainment became a problem. Was it his first big hit — the night of the millennium, when he looked incredulously at the five thousand dollars he had just won with only *one* hand of poker? Was it the day he lost so much money the only way he could cope was to raise the stakes, hoping he could win it all back? At some point, his hundred-dollar bets had become thousand-dollar gambles. His friends and his girlfriend faded from his attention. How did all this happen?

Mark promised himself a special Las Vegas holiday on his thirtieth birthday. He craved the supernatural fairyland feel of Las Vegas. He recalls sitting enchanted, nose pressed to the plane window, at the view of the looming neon signs as the plane touched the runway. That first trip was pure bliss.

More trips followed. Months of playing became years, but eventually the glamour faded. After four years at the casinos, he found himself dipping into his savings, taking out a line of credit to pay for his debts.

During these trips, Mark was also developing a worrisome pattern of eating and drinking colossal amounts of food and alcohol. At first, it seemed to fit with the whole gambling package. Gulping down a twenty-four-ounce cup of soda, he would drive with a mammoth steak cradled on his lap and huge chunks of pie or bags of candy piled in the passenger seat beside him. When he got back to the hotel, he ate even more. Hard liquor replaced soda.

Mark's dissatisfaction intensified. He was losing money too frequently and was facing grave health issues like diabetes and hypertension. He couldn't believe that in his midthirties he had these conditions typical of middle age. Mark stopped gambling for a couple of years, but was back at it one week after a relationship breakup. The lure of the poker and buffet tables was too strong to resist whenever he felt depressed and rejected.

Finally, Mark hit bottom. Early one morning, a trailer park attendant found Mark in his car, soiled in his sweat and urine, literally baking in the August heat of the desert. He had blacked out in a diabetic coma; his phone was bleating incessantly by his side. His office was calling him about an urgent work issue.

Today, Mark is still baffled how he got from the Strip to the far suburbs of Vegas where he was found. He simply can't remember. He guesses that after hours of downing energy-drink chasers, along with eight thousand calories of buffet food, he must have miscalculated his diabetic medication and put himself into a hypoglycemic coma. The sobering fact is that he could have died. Mark stopped gambling for good. He also stopped drinking, realizing that without gambling, he had no desire to drink.

But his eating did not stop.

Mark gorged even more on buffets and roadside takeout. No longer focusing on his gambling, all he thought about was food. In a typical night, while watching the food network, Mark could eat twenty-five to fifty chicken wings, or a large pizza and a rack of ribs, or pulled pork sandwiches. He added litres of soda pop to swallow the volume of food. At the end of the night, he ate more: chips, crackers, and pastries. It was not unusual for him to have a second dinner. He smiles bemusedly, calling this his "nightcap" of prosciutto and huge hunks of cheese on top of a crust of oiled bread. Another late-night snack was his version of an Oreo cookie: an entire box of chocolate chip cookies, generously dipped in butter. We laugh as Mark recalls these memories; we are two food addicts identifying the absurdity of our excesses.

Always interested in cooking, Mark was also excessive in his purchases of food magazines and cookbooks. He bought them by the dozens. By the end of a year, he had accumulated over two hundred cookbooks. "I didn't even notice the shift of attention," he says. And why would he? He was still on a high, having merely shifted his attention from gambling to food. It was a seamless transition.

With dismay, Mark observed he was constantly outgrowing his wardrobe. His doctor's visits were equally alarming to him, with a new diagnosis frightening him at each appointment. One visit he was told he had diabetes, the next hypertension, gout.… The irony was that he was sicker than his father, who was thirty years older than him. But it was the number on the scale of his doctor's office that petrified him the most. Three hundred and four pounds! Through the corner of his eyes he watched the doctor tick off the "morbidly obese" box. His heart thumped. Would his weight gain *ever* stop?

The next week he shoved his leg into a forty-eight-inch size pant leg at the tailor. He pushed harder, but his leg could not fit through, despite repeated tugging at the waistband. These were the pants he had ordered only *three months before*. He gasped. "Now I have to wear fifty-inch pants?" He toppled out of the store. Sitting in his car, tears streaming down his face, he asked himself repeatedly, "How did it come to this?"

Mark joined a commercial weight-loss program for men the next day. In six months, he had quit soda, chips, wings, burgers, even sugar. "Eat crap, get fat," was his favorite motto. His weight dropped over a hundred pounds, and his diabetes improved. He parked his CPAP machine for good and no longer takes medication for high blood pressure.

Mark intuitively knew he had to stop eating sugar, but like so many sugar addicts, he wants to test the waters every now and then. He admits ruefully that whenever he tries to reintroduce sugar or other "kryptonite" foods, he ends up on a massive eating binge. To illustrate, he tells me that last year he ate one Nanaimo bar at a buffet. Since it was a public gathering with others standing shoulder to shoulder, he reasoned it was safe to taste "just one." Surely, he could control any niggling urge to eat just one more. By the end of the night, he discovered to his horror that he had eaten the whole plate.

Today, Mark belongs to a men's group in Toronto. It is a group of about fifty men (and their partners) who meet weekly for education and support. It is an example of how the community can together, grassroots style, combat the lures of our toxic food environment. Mark says his membership in the group is the main reason why he is still sober and has maintained his hundred-pound weight loss. His recovery work with them has kept his addictive urges in check so that the food obsessions do not return or morph into some new obsession. He knows that he is an addict, just waiting for the new fix.

How to Stop the Bouncing Ball

The brain chemistry that drives the addict to seek pleasure beyond the point of satiety is similar, whether the user favours Jack Daniels or Jack-in-the-Box. So what's an addict to do? Is it possible that, even after years of working at treating one's primary addiction, one is never safe from this monster disease?

Yes, this is often true, but I have good news: there is hope.

First, just knowing that you are at risk is enormously helpful. The scientific understanding and cultural acceptance of addiction as a *disease* that exists today can help an individual resist trading one addiction for another. Unlike the unknowing early members of Alcoholics Anonymous, who suggested that eating sweets was the best way to treat the craving for booze, we now know where that can lead — right to the nearest Sugar Mountain aisle.[1] "As an alcoholic *and* a food addict,

I got really resentful at AA members who told me to have ice cream whenever I wanted to drink," says a woman in recovery. "They just didn't get it."

Those well-intentioned old-timers were counselling newer members to disregard out-of-control eating and weight gain because they were lesser evils. Food, they said, would not do the same damage that their previous drug did. And they were right: switching an addiction from alcohol to sugar is an effective *short-term* strategy for giving up alcohol … until the long-term consequences kick in.

Many members of Overeaters Anonymous and Food Addicts Anonymous, in fact, have come to these fellowships after many years of sobriety from alcohol. They have finally recognized that their addictive impulses have merely shifted. They have realized that they are reacting to food just as they reacted to alcohol or other drugs, with little or no control. And the consequences are just as potentially deadly.

For such cross-addicted persons, I believe it is best to eventually stop all addictions. Doing so forces the addict to treat the addictive impulse rather than merely transferring it from one substance to another. But in order to prevent the phenomenon of switched addictions, more work needs to be done. This is the difference between being what's known as a "wet drunk" and a "dry drunk." The dry drunk has put down her drug and so is no longer "wet." However, she is still a drunk, with all the behaviours and maladapted attitudes that will lead her into another addiction, or possibly into a relapse back to her primary addiction.

"I was suffering from untreated alcoholism, even though I was sober," says Teresa. "I was sleeping around, spending money like crazy, and behaving worse than I did when I was drinking. Just staying off the booze did not take care of the real problem, which was *me*."

Once the drug was put away, Teresa needed to work on dealing with her real problems, which were her self-destructive ways of coping with life. "I hadn't had a drink for more than twenty years," says Fred, another addict, from New England, "but I was ready to either drink or put a gun to my head. I sure wasn't happy." Fred says he never really enjoyed any peace of mind until he began working on his attitude, his way of looking at life.

These people, like so many, required an attitude adjustment if they were to find serenity or peace of mind. Most will achieve this serenity once they have begun to practice crucial coping skills like admitting wrongdoing, forgiving others, and learning to tolerate the trials and tribulations of life — what is known as "life on life's terms" — with equanimity. It is this type of therapeutic work that makes the difference between achieving *food abstinence,* in which the trigger foods are eliminated but the person is still craving, and *food serenity,* in which the need for food, or any other substitute, has dissipated in the face of other, more fulfilling experiences.

Want to stay clear of the trigger foods and be happy too? The last chapter of this book will address how to achieve this. I will also describe what I believe are the key ingredients to a good life after the food has been shelved. You will meet Martha, who has crossed that great divide from food addiction to food serenity, and hear how she has found peace of mind. Her story will show you that freedom from food addiction can really taste great.

CHAPTER SIXTEEN

FREEDOM TASTES GREAT!
FINDING FOOD SERENITY

Alcoholics Anonymous did not begin when Bill Wilson got sober. It began[1] when Wilson met Bob Smith and the two shared their stories. Like so many other people struggling with addiction, Bill Wilson was very good at getting sober; the problem was *staying* sober. It's hard to face life "stark raving abstinent." Put down your drug, and then what? How does one face the night without that trusted friend: the tub of ice cream or the box of jelly doughnuts? All the emotions, from self-loathing to boredom, crowd in, making sobriety a miserable experience. And after addicts have completed detox, when these feelings are most intense, they are left with their feelings and no drug to placate their pain.

When Bill picked up the phone one fateful night, which historians claim spawned AA, he was struggling with sobriety in its most painfully raw form. He understood that he could not stay sober without help. Although he *knew* that drinking was not the answer to his turmoil, his need to relieve his pain was overwhelming. He called another alcoholic who would sympathize with his irrational desire to drink again. Dr. Bob, who would become co-founder of the largest self-help movement of the twentieth century, answered the phone. He listened, but did not know what to say to relieve Bill's anguish. To the amazement of them both, that was not necessary. For Bill to stay sober that night, it was enough that he talked to someone who understood.

The Spiritual Challenge of Abstinence

Service for the benefit of another addict is one of the most important ingredients in staying sober from any addiction. This is evident in the stories of many of the recovered food addicts we have met in this book: Phil, Susan, Harvey, Tony, me.

The single most important tool toward lasting success, however, seems to be a relationship with a higher power. For many, unfortunately, this is also the biggest obstacle to attending one of the twelve-step groups.

The emphasis on spirituality is often why people turn away at the doors of a twelve-step meeting. When I have recommended such programs to clients, many respond, "I don't believe in God or a higher power or all that spiritual stuff." If the word "spiritual" does not sit well with you, try "psychological wellness" or sense of "inner self." It is this spiritual (not religious) dimension of the twelve-step groups, complemented with their fellowship, that is the added reason members claim they are able to remain abstinent over the long term. Recovered addicts will say that eventually they *had to* succumb to some kind of belief in *something* outside of themselves. They had to trust there was a strength — anything — to help them stop killing themselves with food. Time and again, they saw that they could not succeed by relying on their own willpower. Eventually, a personal crisis, shifting priorities, a difficult social situation, or even boredom would take over and before they knew it, they would be bingeing again. To avoid that, they found that they needed a particular kind of support; they needed to believe in something that was beyond where they were currently stuck.

The book of Alcoholics Anonymous was written in 1939 when religious language was normal discourse for that time. Therefore, twelve-step literature reflects this in its common use of "God-language." Many twelve-step members use the word God as a kind of shorthand for the "higher power" that helped them when their own resources were not sufficient. The twelve-step program, however, does not stress religion, per se, it emphasizes spirituality. The fellowship is intended to be secular in nature and has been able to welcome everyone from atheists to religious fundamentalists. Spiritual, not religious, their only goal is to fill the void that eliminating food has left behind with comfort, grace, and hope.

For the recovering food addict, a spiritual practice can mean something as simple as discussing your daily food choices with someone. There is a strength (power) in this action that is greater than what she was doing without such support. In twelve-step language, this daily routine is known as "surrendering your food" to a sponsor or a "food buddy." Other examples of spiritual practices are meditating, reading enlightening literature, or doing volunteer work. Members are encouraged to adopt a practice of asking for help with both abstinence *and* life events each morning and saying, "thank you" (which produces serotonin) for managing to stay abstinent at the end of each day. A person does not have to believe in God or *any* deity for this practice to be effective.

Martha: Freedom Tastes Great!

"Gratitude," Martha says, looking at me with tears wet on her cheeks. Holding her hands to her face as if in supplication, she says, "I live in a constant state of gratitude. I'm grateful for my health. I can garden now. I can walk my dog. I can work."

I am sitting at a large kitchen table in Martha's farmhouse. There is a big black dog lying on its side in the small cold room separating the kitchen from the doorway. I am typing on my laptop as Martha speaks, stirring her tea.

Martha is a sixty-year-old woman who can boast over thirty years of food sobriety. She stands five-feet-two-inches tall and her current weight is 135 pounds, giving her a BMI just shy of 25. This places her in the "normal" category, a standing that is in stark contrast with that of thirty years ago when she reached her top weight of 245 pounds.[2] At that time, she would have been classified as morbidly obese. She has been abstinent from sugar and flour since 1988.

I learned about Martha from a colleague who had told me about a therapist who worked with food addicts. That caught my interest — there was someone who actually treated people with food addictions? That therapist was Martha. She had introduced my colleague to a group of other food addicts, many of whom had achieved long-term recovery.

I was especially eager to meet Martha when she said that she had maintained her weight loss for years *and* was happy. The two just didn't seem to go hand-in-hand with most of the people I was meeting at that time. I drove ninety minutes west of Toronto into rural farmland to visit Martha. Her office is on the first floor of a red-brick farmhouse that sits just outside the sleepy town of Hagersville. I remembered this town because several years earlier a huge stack of tires in the local dump had caught fire. The smoke had smouldered for weeks, with dark clouds of dust drifting for miles into neighbouring cities. It had been the source of alarm for environmentalists and the focus of regular television clips.

Martha has a steady private practice, with clients who drive in from Windsor, London, and Hamilton to see her. Along with her one-on-one therapy, she runs food addiction and trauma groups as well as after-care meetings on weekends. For those, clients will often come early to spend the night in her large house before the group starts the next day. She has even hosted food addiction therapist Kay Sheppard from the United States on several occasions. She and another long-term food addict also maintain a twelve-step peer support group of food addicts.

Martha is a pleasant woman with bright eyes and an easy grin. Wearing a sleeveless print shirt, navy shorts, and light blue flip-flops, she exudes energy — I have seen her bound up a flight of stairs, carrying a box of kitchen utensils in one hand and two stacking chairs in the other. Leaning forward enthusiastically, she tells her story.

Her earliest memory is climbing onto the counter in the family kitchen at the age of four. She yanked out the cake supplies — the brown sugar, chocolate chips, and the flour, and ate everything at once. "I was already lying about my food," she says. "I stole money from my father for candy." In grade school, she was the chubbiest kid in her class. This was during the 1960s, she reminds me, when childhood obesity was unusual. Most kids were lean and ran through the schoolyard without a thought. Not her. She was teased mercilessly and would go home crying. Her doctor put her on diet pills, which worked — until she stopped taking them.

She abhorred diets. She remembers an aunt who would not let her eat her candy until she was leaving to go home. "If I was good," Martha recalls, "she gave me *one* cookie! It was hell! I always wanted more!"

During her college years, she took to drinking alcohol as well as eating even more compulsively. She found a neighbour who ate as she did and they became "binge buddies," going out together to buffets and sharing baked goods.

After finishing school, she became a teacher of home economics, which meant that she could taste her students' food projects. Later, she worked in the restaurant industry, developing menus and taste-testing new recipes on a daily basis. Food became her life. Her weight soared, and she reached nearly 250 pounds as she binged and drank her way through her twenties and early thirties.

Having watched her father die of alcoholism, Martha feared she was heading in the same direction until, sometime in the mid-1980s, she heard about AA and decided to stop drinking. After that, she ate even more. Gradually, she started to see that her eating was just as out of control as her drinking had been. When someone in an AA meeting admitted they also went to OA, Martha knew what she had to do next.

It was in the OA meetings[3] that she heard about other people who obsessed about their food the way she did. They also ate too much, ate in secret, stole food. Even when they were sick of what they were eating, they ate. Martha could relate to almost every "share" she heard.

While at the meetings, she learned the techniques that some members were using to manage their weight. She liked to eat "male-sized" portions instead of the recommended smaller, "female-sized" portions because they made her feel more satisfied. She would run for hours to control her weight so she could accommodate her larger portions and the occasional slips from her rigid diet. At OA, however, Martha learned that some people purged and used laxatives to control their weight.

Ruefully, she admits, "I did not hear the recovery in the messages of the people sharing. Instead, I learned how to vomit and how many laxatives I would need to lose weight." New tools in hand, Martha was able to reduce her weight to 107 pounds. Ironically, she developed anorexia while in OA.

Her sponsor finally intervened and told Martha that being thin did not mean she was healthy. Her eating behaviour, her focus on food and weight, and her irritability and unhappy moods were all signs of an unhealthy program. But what could Martha do? Were there only two choices? Gaining weight again or being thin and miserable? Luckily for her, she found the book that would change her life. One day, a contact at work asked her to review a book called *Food Addiction: The Body Knows*, by Kay Sheppard. It literally changed her life.

Sheppard's book told her she had a food addiction. She realized that sugar and flour were problems for her; whenever she ate them she couldn't stop. She had a hunch that she was "addicted," because she recognized that the way she ate sugar was the same as the way she used to drink. But was it possible that she was actually *addicted* to these foods and that to escape the addiction it would be necessary for her to follow a plan that removed these — as if they were drugs — from her diet? She could not believe that anyone would actually suggest this. Still, in desperation, she decided to try Kay Sheppard's food plan as it was laid out in the book. No sugar, no flour, no grains, and she found that weighing and measuring her food was also a useful precaution.

Although she initially suffered withdrawal from her junk foods, she found that, within weeks, she lost her cravings to eat them. She no longer felt the obsession to binge or had to plan her days or social visits around her meals. As long as she kept to her food plan, she maintained a steady weight and, at the same time, felt quite sane about her eating behaviour.

Martha discovered, however, that support from others was crucial. Being accountable to another person about her food choices made it easier to deal with those pesky thoughts that kept taunting her — "Just try a small bite of *this*," or "Just have a quick taste of *that*."

Years went by in stable recovery. She ate well, even reintroducing some foods like grains back into her diet. She kept her weight at an even

120 pounds. Martha was confident about her approach and wanted to share her experience. She decided to treat food addicts, especially when she saw how some of her trauma clients were abusing food in the same way that she once had.

Then menopause hit. This was harder than Martha expected. She became moody and her sleep was disrupted. To her dismay, she started to gain weight. Even though her diet did not change, her weight crept back up, rising from 120 to 135 to 150 pounds. She became worried.

Beyond eating richer foods and doing less exercise, which is typical of middle age, there are other biological reasons why women gain weight at this time in their life. Menopause occurs because ovulation stops, resulting in less production of estrogen. Animal studies have indicated that estrogen plays a role in the metabolic rate; reduced estrogen results in the body burning calories at a slower pace.

Lower estrogen also seems to predispose women to insulin resistance, which, as we have seen in previous chapters, increases the likelihood of stronger food cravings and weight gain. As estrogen drops, the ratio of estrogen to testosterone shifts so that there is more testosterone available to negatively affect women. Findings from the study of Women's Health Across the Nation (SWAN) of more than 350 women between the ages of forty-two and sixty showed that increased levels of bio-available testosterone led to an increase in visceral fat, leading to metabolic syndrome, arthritis, depression, and even Alzheimer's. This study[4] presents the most accurate understanding to date about the origin and dangers of "middle age spread." Sobering news indeed.

When Martha broke her wrist during her menopause period, she could no longer exercise or work in her garden. Her weight edged up higher, to 170 pounds. Now she was really desperate. What to do? She felt that her food plan, which had worked for many years, had turned against her. Why was it not working now? She had no idea that hormones could have such a great impact on her physical and mental stability.

The worst, she explained to me, was that she was sure others questioned her abstinence. Why else would she be gaining weight again? She was tempted to restrict her calories but knew that this could threaten her abstinence. She was sure she had to change her diet somehow but felt that if she altered her food plan she would be "breaking the rules" of her program. Was this just her food-addled brain speaking, tempting her to stray from her plan?

After some deliberation, Martha decided to experiment with her food plan. Again, she stopped eating grains; instead, she supplemented her meals with more vegetables. She had science backing her up on this: given that grains are higher on the glycemic index than most green and brown vegetables, she would be eating fewer starches that would rapidly metabolize into sugar and from there become abdominal fat.

Eating fewer grains had worked for her years before. She hoped that doing so again would once more help her to reduce her weight. There might be another benefit, too. Martha was convinced that, because of her family's history of celiac disease, she might be allergic to wheat. Now in menopause, without the protective shield of estrogen, this gluten allergy became apparent. As it turned out, this small tweak of removing the wheat — and the gluten in the wheat — from her diet made all the difference.

Lyn-Genet Recitas's book *The Plan* suggests that people who *do* eat nutritious foods but still gain weight should make the effort to determine which foods could be allergens. She posits that simply being allergic to specific foods might be the reason for persistent weight gain (through the inflammatory response, which can lead to weight gain, arthritis, even diabetes) and recommends an elimination diet to identify the hidden culprit.[5] The gluten in wheat is an obvious choice to eliminate, since many people develop a gluten allergy later in life.

Martha did more than change her diet, though. She learned how stress and a lack of sleep contribute to obesity, so she focused on developing a healthy sleep schedule and started doing regular yoga for stress relief. She stopped her long-distance running and other cardio-related exercises. Instead, she switched to weight-bearing exercises that did not involve the surges of adrenaline and cortisone, both of which she believed were contributing to her gradual weight gain. Soon her weight dropped and stabilized at its current level of 135 pounds. She felt better: her mood improved, she was sleeping again, and she felt more emotionally stable.

Today, Martha's ingredients for sobriety are simple: she follows a plan based on stress management, good sleep, and an abstinent diet. She has learned that an abstinent diet that has worked for many years may need to be tweaked due to age and hormonal changes. While the general principles of no sugar and no flour still apply, a food plan needs to be adapted to the unique needs of the food addict.

Despite the importance of an abstinent diet, Martha believes that the key ingredient to her long-term recovery is her spiritual condition. This has become more important to her than her weight or her diet. She knows that she could not follow her food plan without the broader perspective that a peaceful spiritual condition affords. It keeps her doubts, emotional upsets, and hormonal changes at bay.

Gardening, walking her dog, and working are all spiritual acts that she relishes to maintain her sobriety. These activities give her waves of gratitude that sustain her through the tougher moments of any day. "I am in constant prayer through the day," she says to me as I type vigorously on my laptop. She beams with what I can only call a look of serenity as she gazes over her farmland though the window behind me.

EPILOGUE: A HAPPY ENDING, ONE DAY AT A TIME

In the spring of 2013, the struggle with food was back. Did I really think it had gone away?

The impact was startling. I looked at the tablespoon of almond butter and felt a surge of warmth and excitement. After the third tablespoon, I groaned and put the jar away. I knew I was in trouble. I had been here before and I could feel the dread beneath the exhilaration.

The next day I picked up the nut butter jar and morosely stared at it. Then, despite my misgivings, I ate three more tablespoons. But I hardly noticed the taste or the size of my servings (each heaping spoonful hovered at about 1.5 tablespoons). The old chorus had already started: *Why not savour just one more spoonful? Just one more to really taste the delicious sweetness of the nuts, the succulent smoothness of the texture?* I managed to confine myself that day to only those three mouthfuls, but I wanted more.

The next day I barely restrained myself, eating five towering tablespoons. I knew even this would not suffice. It was as if an old hunger had resurrected itself, a hunger that seemed bottomless, impossible to satisfy. I was in a vortex of addiction that Dr. Gabor Maté has described as the "realm of the hungry ghosts."[1] This had nothing to do with taste anymore; I was trying to get a feeling of satisfaction again that was becoming more elusive the more I tried to get it. After a month, I was sometimes shovelling more than ten mammoth table-spoons into my mouth each night. I knew I had to stop, but each night I gave in. I just had to revel in the sweetness and the smooth, creamy texture.

The scale became a terror. After noticing the first few extra pounds, I promised myself I would stop once I gained five. Then it was ten. The scale kept climbing as my binges continued. By the time the scale indicated that I had gained fifteen extra pounds, I knew I needed a new strategy. I planned to cut back my nut butter splurges to only once a week, just on Saturdays. I reserved cashew butter for special occasions. That plan lasted three days. I couldn't possibly hold out until the weekend.

So I went back to devising how to eat only a few tablespoons a day. I asked my partner to monitor me, parcelling out the tablespoons so I could not cheat. That didn't last for even one day; I simply could not bring myself to ask her. I scanned my options — what rule could I devise that might actually work?

To stop eating this highly triggering food that had trapped me in my current insane web of obsession and denial, craving and despair, did not seem possible. I could not put out of my mind the memory of that first night, when I savoured the first tablespoon of almond butter and felt that glow, as if an inner light had flicked on. The thoughts in my head kept leaping from *How could a food do this?* to *I can't give this up, this is just too good to give up. I want that buzz, just one more time.*

Why was I here, at this place, again? Why, when I — an addiction clinician! — understood exactly what was happening and actually knew how to stop this cycle, was I caught in this loop again?

It took one year before I was ready to take the only action I knew would work. One year because I was stubborn and unwilling to give up the memory of that first night, wanting it back, if even for a few minutes. I could not let go of the anticipation that the next tablespoon would again give me that sparkle of delight. Nothing else I knew of could give me that thrill, other than alcohol, which I had foresworn five years earlier. Finally, I threw up my hands in despair. Sure, nuts are healthy, but, in my hands, they're also dangerous.

Using the only strategy that would work, I grudgingly admitted to myself that I had a problem with this particular food: nut butters were a trigger, so I had to quit eating them forever. I already knew I could not eat sugar, bread, chips, and pasta. Now I had to admit that I was powerless to control my use of nuts, too. The only solution: abstinence. Some weeks later, I discovered once again the truth about eating trigger foods: I would do anything — fast for an entire day or walk for hours to burn calories — just to allow myself to eat them. The craving was that strong. But, once I stop, my desire gradually fades; it is as if the beast inside me is deflating each day that I deny it fuel. Slowly, I lose the mental obsession and regain my peace of mind. It took me four years to lose the fifteen pounds I gained, but I did stop the disease that had caught me off guard once I willingly surrendered to the solution.

Why am I telling you this at the end of *Food Junkies*, when I should be offering hope of freedom from addiction? My intention is to instill hope, but within a realistic context. Based on my personal and clinical experience, I believe that addiction of any kind has no cure. There is only a daily reprieve from its course of malignant action. The engine is always idling; all it needs is a foot on the gas pedal.

It perplexes me that as knowledgeable as I am about this issue, I can still succumb to my addiction. Despite knowing the answer, I still naively ask myself: *Will this ever go away? Will my desire to eat my trigger foods always be there, ready to vex me at any weak moment? Surely I can stop if I really want to, can't I? Can I really be addicted to food like a drug addict to a drug?*

The evidence has shown me, however, time and again, even to this day, that I am still a food addict. As I hope I have demonstrated in the many examples provided in this book, food addicts are always in recovery, always just one mouthful away from the next binge. Admitting we are addicts is not about holding onto a "victim" identity and wallowing in despair. It is simply a reminder that we are powerless over our internal urges, cravings, and addictions once they are triggered. It is our job to be sure that we identify and avoid the triggers in the first place.

It is our job to avoid the first bite.

I continue to work in this field of addiction, knowing that helping others corrals my inner addict. Communicating the scientific information and the clinical scenarios that I have included in this book to illustrate the power of food addiction is of great benefit to me personally. Like everyone else, I need to be reminded that this urge inside me is bigger than my intellect, my scientific knowledge, and my will. I hear the message every time I help others; the words are meant as much for me as for my patients. I, too, need to hear the message repeatedly so that it sinks in, one day at a time.

Full circle. Many years ago, as a teenager, I was stealing food from hapless nursing home residents, starting on a journey through the dark, hungry side within. I did not know what this urge to eat was about or how to manage the power of my compulsions. Today, I deal with the same impulses, but with clarity and purpose. I can take the energy from the cravings and propel myself instead to do meaningful work, with and for others. When I do this, my story has a happy ending.

My message to you is that if you have a hunger that seems eternally ravenous, there is an explanation. You may be a food addict. Once you understand why this peculiar phenomenon of desiring food beyond "normal" hunger occurs, the solution to quelling that need is obvious. It cannot be done by filling that seemingly bottomless pit with food and more food; this strategy, as no doubt many of you have already discovered, does not create the satisfaction for which you are longing. The solution to quenching that insatiable hunger is to put the alluring food down, since eating more of it only leads to wanting more of it.

A relentless, inescapable want.

Rather than trying to receive gratification from food or any other addictive substance, turning that desire toward connecting with others placates that ache. By virtue of being human, we all have the need to be in relationships. By sharing our humanity, we can bond with others and feed our own soul. We are then able to feel full at last; the bottomless pit of addiction can then fade like a bad dream.

With this added effort of extending ourselves beyond our "quick fix," food no longer stands in the way of connection. Food sobriety can become food serenity. Freedom from food obsession can taste better than anything you could possibly imagine.

I invite you to leave the bleak world of food junkies and join me, by helping others on this journey toward food serenity. The power is ours.

ACKNOWLEDGEMENTS

I have many thanks to give for this book that has been a dream come true.

First, I must acknowledge my appreciation to Phil Werdell, my colleague, who led the way in unearthing and compiling the research for the first edition of this book. Your thinking about food addiction, as well as your clinical work and advocacy in the field, is unmatched. I credit you for putting the field of food addiction on the map. While the second edition moves into territory separate from your work, much of my essential thinking comes from your fundamental contributions. You are the giant upon whose shoulders I stand.

I wish to express my gratitude to Dundurn Press for taking a chance on this audacious topic. There is a great reluctance amongst many to acknowledge addiction of any sort, especially food addiction. It is only by having the willingness to take a stand that it becomes possible for the many affected to change their lives and make the crucial transition to health. I am thankful to Dominic Farrell for the editorial finishing touches, Courtney Horner for the design, and, finally, the marketing department for their assistance. All of you have allowed me to make this the best book possible for this subject at this time.

Hilary McMahon, a special thank you for believing in my vision and for your persistence in helping me find a venue for this message. I would also like to thank Anne Collins and Ann Dowsett Johnston. I am indebted to you for your early encouragement and editorial suggestions, as well as for your sound wisdom regarding the publishing industry today.

I am indebted to Christine Palmer for the nuts-and-bolts research, and David Hayes and David Kilgour, for your writing and editorial aplomb. This book would have been impossible to read without all of you. Chris, you helped untie the many layers of food addiction and made the voluminous research manageable. Your insights and writing showed me how to present the clinical and medical information in a readable format. I am indebted to your vision and personal commitment to the food addiction field. David Kilgour and David Hayes, I thank both of you for your steadfast and calm manner as you brought the book together in its final form.

Esther Helga Guðmundsdóttir, you are a model of food addiction recovery and a leader in food addiction advocacy. Your program in Iceland was the first of its kind and remains a stellar example of how food addiction services can be provided. Your new work to educate clinicians about food addiction treatment ensures quality and consistency on an international basis. I hope that this book sparks advances toward many more such services as yours.

A special thank you to Martha Peirce for being a pioneer in food addiction advocacy and food addiction counselling services in Canada. I thank you for having the courage to tell your story in this book, and for your tireless endeavours. We are finally coming out of the "dark ages." Renae Norton, I wish to acknowledge your willingness to step outside of your profession and speak the truth about food addiction as it relates to eating disorders. Such professional courage, which challenges the prevailing psychological beliefs around eating disorders, has helped many people to better understand their potentially fatal condition and get relief from it. Your clinical insights have especially contributed greatly toward my understanding of the anorexic/bulimic food addict — the bulimorexic.

Tony Vassallo and Sandra Elia, I applaud your efforts on the Canadian front. Tony, you bring the message to the men who might otherwise not make it into the recovery rooms that are populated mainly by women. Sandra, you bring the message of recovery to the bariatric community, which continues to be bombarded with surgical and medical options rather than the message of food addiction.

Many have contributed their stories to this book and are acknowledged here and elsewhere by name. Others, who preferred anonymity — you know who you are — your contributions have been essential. All your stories have helped me present the many guises in which food addiction can appear. Each of your stories will touch someone who is reading this book.

For their scientific leadership, I would like to thank Nora Volkow, Kelly Brownell, Mark Gold, Ernest Noble, Bart Hoebel, Nicole Avena, and Ashley Gearhardt. Their works have all contributed toward helping me translate the science of food addiction into manageable clinical and therapeutic interventions. A special mention to Dr. Robert Lustig for his indefatigable efforts to urge a clinical standard of care that is scientific and unyielding to the forces of our current political and economic climate.

Overeaters Anonymous (OA), Food Addicts Anonymous (FAA), Grey Sheeters Anonymous (GSA), Food Addicts in Recovery Anonymous (FA), Compulsive Eaters Anonymous-HOW (CEA-HOW), Anorexics and Bulimics Anonymous (ABA), and Recovering Food Addicts Anonymous (RFA) have demonstrated that thousands of people can recover from addictive food diseases using the twelve-step model.

I wish to acknowledge my family and friends, for all of your insights and experience. We all endure, on some level, addictive impulses which are so easily provoked by living in our current society. You have all helped me place food addiction within the larger context of human life with its struggles and its redemptive qualities.

A special heartfelt thank you to Lorraine Johnson, who has been with me throughout the early and often lonely years of food addiction advocacy in Canada. You have been a steady companion, offering your organizational skills to my muddle; your willingness to come through at the last minute has made many a project possible and fun. Your encouragement and vision in our cause has been invaluable in the bleaker moments.

I also want to acknowledge Dianne Piaskoski. Your research and proofreading contributions were always quick and incisive, and your spirit helped make our little band of advocates a joy.

I owe a debt of gratitude to Renascent, the treatment centre where I work as Medical Director. In 2016 we pioneered a residential program designed solely for the food addict. Thank you to the many dedicated and skilled members of this organization. I am blessed to have worked side by side with you in this incredible venture. We are building a vibrant Toronto hub of awareness for food addiction, so that others across Canada and beyond may discover that they are no longer alone.

On that note, I would like to thank the many people who have been integral in my own personal peer-support networks: Peter W., Chris D., and the many friends who must remain nameless but are ever-present in my mind. You are the food that feeds my soul.

Finally, I would like to acknowledge Cathy, my life partner. You have been resolute in your time, patience, and encouragement. Your editorial honesty has been painful to hear at times, but always spot on. Your love and support have made every bit of this journey worthwhile. I look forward to many more such adventures in this "happily ever after" life we live together.

NOTES

PREFACE TO THE SECOND EDITION

1) Diet clubs can be informal, ad hoc groups, or organized by large, corporate entities such as Weight Watchers, TOPS, LA Weight Loss, Jenny Craig, or PRISM (Christian) Weight Loss Groups. Diet pills include over-the-counter medications, most of which contain caffeine, and prescription drugs, such as phentermine, an appetite suppressant, and Xenical, a fat absorption blocker. Diet doctors provide pills, shots, and food and exercise regimens. Edible diet supports are less popular today than they were in the sixties, seventies, and eighties, when Ayds, Metrecal, and Carnation Slender were big sellers.

THIS BOOK, BITE SIZE: OUR MESSAGE TO YOU

1) W.C. King, et al., "Prevalence of Alcohol Use Disorders Before and After Bariatric Surgery," *Journal of the American Medical Association* 307, no. 23 (June 20, 2012): 2516–25.

CHAPTER TWO
I JUST LIKE TO EAT! EATING AND OVEREATING

1) To read more about being "wired to enjoy food," see Paul M. Johnson, and Paul J. Kenny, "Dopamine D2 receptors in addiction-like reward dysfunction and compulsive eating in obese rats," *Nature Neuroscience* 13, no. 5 (May 2010): 635–41; D.M. Blumenthal, and M.S. Gold, "Neurobiology of food addiction," *Current Opinion in Clinical Nutrition and Metabolic Care* 13, no. 4 (July 2010): 359–65; and David A. Kessler, *The End of Overeating: Taking Control of the Insatiable American Appetite, Reprint* (Emmaus, PA: Rodale Books, 2010).

2) See P. Sumithran, et al., "Long-Term Persistence of Hormonal Adaptations to Weight Loss," *New England Journal of Medicine* 365, no. 17 (October 27, 2011): 1597–604, for a fascinating discussion of the interplay of hormones and weight.

3) See Stephen C. Woods, "Gastrointestinal Satiety Signals I: An overview of gastrointestinal signals that influence food intake," *Journal of Physiology: Gastrointestinal and Liver Physiology* 286, no. 1 (January 2004): G7–13.

4) Prader-Willi: Basic information about this childhood obesity-causing disease is available from the Foundation for Prader-Willi Research: www.fpwr.org.

5) Alexandra Shapiro, et al., "Fructose-induced leptin resistance exacerbates weight gain in response to subsequent high-fat feeding," *American Journal of Physiology: Regulatory, Integrative and Comparative Physiology* 295, no. 5 (November 2008): R1370–75.

6) Luigia Cristino, et al., "Obesity-driven synaptic remodeling affects endocannabinoid control of orexinergic neurons," *Proceedings of the National Academy of Sciences of the United States of America* 110, no. 24 (June 11, 2013): E2229–38.

7) For more information about leptin resistance and to get a proposed diet plan that follows this theory, see http://jackkruse.com/my-leptin-prescription/.

8) For more information about leptin resistance and to get a proposed diet, see Stephen Phinney and Jeff Volek, *The Art and Science of Low Carbohydrate Living* (2011).

CHAPTER THREE
SUGAR MAKES ME HAPPY!

1) Ann D'Adamo, "U.S. Weight Loss and Diet Trends 2016-2017," Women's Marketing, www.womensmarketing.com/blog/u.s.-weight -loss-and-diet-trends-2016-wmi.

2) Harriet Brown, "The Weight of the Evidence: It's Time to Stop Telling Fat People to Become Thin," Slate, www.slate.com/articles/health_ and_science/medical_examiner/2015/03/diets_do_not_work_the_ thin_evidence_that_losing_weight_makes_you_healthier.html.

CHAPTER FOUR
SO, WHAT EXACTLY IS FOOD ADDICTION?

1) For more information about the limbic system and details that explain the physiology of the human brain, see www.brainanatomy. net. The limbic system is composed of the ventral tegmental area, the nucleus accumbens, and the frontal lobe. Its job is to direct our moods, motivations, and unconscious instinctual behaviours toward survival-enhancing functions.

2) See Loretta Graziano Breuning, *Meet Your Happy Chemicals* (N.p: System Integrity Press, 2012) for a fun discussion of these "happy" neurochemicals.

3) This phrase can be found in "Reflections on Ice Breaking," a poem by American writer and humorist, Frederic Ogden Nash (1902–1971).

4) See discussion of the fermentation of natural fruit and alcohol content in Michael Pollan, *Cooked* (New York: Penguin Press, 2013).

5) These figures come from four graphs that give a comparison of dopamine release (a mean percent of the basal output of four rats) in response to four popular drugs of abuse. See Gaetano di Chiara and Assunta Imperato, "Drugs abused by humans preferentially increase synaptic dopamine concentrations in the mesolimbic system of freely moving rats," *Proceedings of the National Academy of Sciences of the United States of America* 84, no. 14 (July 1988): 5274–78.

6) David J. Linden is the author of *The Compass of Pleasure: How Our Brains Make Fatty Foods, Orgasm, Exercise, Marijuana, Generosity, Vodka, Learning, and Gambling Feel So Good* (New York: Viking,

2011). He was interviewed on National Public Radio's *Fresh Air* in June 2011. The title of the episode was "Compass of Pleasure: Why Some Things Feel So Good."

7) See Maia Szalavitz, "Can Eating Junk Food Really Be an Addiction?" *Time*, last modified April 03, 2010, http://content.time.com/time/health/article/0,8599,1977604,00. html. See also, P.M. Johnson, and P.J. Kenny, "Dopamine D2 receptors in addiction-like reward dysfunction and compulsive eating in obese rats," *Nature Neuroscience* 13, no. 5 (2010): 635–41.

8) See Adam Drewnowski et al., "Naloxone, an opiate blocker, reduces the consumption of sweet high-fat foods in obese and lean female binge eaters," *American Journal of Clinical Nutrition* 61, no. 6 (1995): 1206–12.

9) Bartley G. Hoebel, a Princeton University professor (1935–2011) conducted early research on an area of the brain called the hypothalamus and its control of eating and satiety. For his signature study, see Nicole Avena, et al., "Evidence for sugar addiction: Behavioural and neurochemical effects of intermittent, excessive sugar intake," *Neuroscience and Biobehavioral Reviews* 32, no. 1 (2008): 20–39. See also Nicole Avena, and Bartley G. Hoebel, "A diet promoting sugar dependency causes behavioral cross-sensitization to a low dose of amphetamine," *Neuroscience* 122, no. 1 (2003): 17–20. This key study suggested that bingeing on sugar could lead to increased sensitivity to amphetamine, possibly due to a lasting alteration in the dopamine system. See also C.H. Wideman, "Implications of an Animal Model of Sugar Addiction, Withdrawal, and Relapse for Human Health," *Nutritional Neuroscience* 8, no. 5–6 (2005): 269–76, which deals primarily with demonstrations of sugar addiction in rats; and Nicole M. Avena, "Sugar-dependent rats show enhanced intake of unsweetened ethanol," *Alcohol* 34 (2004): 203–9. By demonstrating the cross sensitivity involving alcohol and sugar addictions we can interpret there is a common addictive dynamic between both.

10) See "The Family Afterward" in *Alcoholics Anonymous* (New York: Alcoholics Anonymous World Services, 2001). This chapter notes

twice that eating sweets — at least in 1939 — was an acceptable and *recommended* way to stave off a craving for alcohol.

11) See Science Daily for a discussion of review of the Scripps study that showed that food and overeating can be addictive for rodents and by implication for people.

12) See Pedro Rada et al., "A High-Fat meal, or Intraperitoneal Administration of a Fat Emulsion, Increases Extracellular Dopamine in the Nucleus Accumbens," *Brain Sciences* 2, no. 2 (June 11, 2012): 242–53.

13) MRI and PET are abbreviations for *magnetic resonance imaging* and *positron emission tomography*, respectively. MRIs allow radiologists to see inside some areas of the body that cannot be seen otherwise. PET is a technique that produces a three-dimensional image or picture of functional processes in the body. Researchers have used these tools to study addiction: See N.D. Volkow et al., "Cocaine Addiction: Hypothesis Derived from Imaging Studies with PET," *Journal of Addictive Diseases* 15, no. 4 (February 1996): 55–71.

14) Gene-Jack Wang et al., "Similarity Between Obesity and Drug Addiction as Assessed by Neurofunctional Imaging: A Concept Review," *Journal of Addictive Diseases* 23 (2004): 39–53. See also, P.K. Thanos, "Food restriction markedly increases dopamine D2 receptor (D2R) in a rat model of obesity as assessed with in-vivo muPET imaging," *Synapse* 62, no.1 (January 2008): 50–61; and E.P. Noble et al., "D2 dopamine receptor gene and obesity," *International Journal of Eating Disorders* 15 (1994): 205–17.

15) Manjula Puthenedam, "PET imaging shows fewer dopamine receptors in drug addicts," *Health Imaging*, last modified April 28, 2010, www.healthimaging.com/topics/molecular-imaging/study-pet-imaging-shows-fewer-dopamine-receptors-drug-addicts.

16) See N.D. Volkow, G.-J. Wang, D. Tomasi, and R.D. Baler, "Pro v Con Reviews: Is Food Addictive? Obesity and Addiction: Neurobiological Overlaps," *Obesity Reviews* 14 no. 1 (2013) 2-18, and *Current Psychiatry Reports* December 2015, 17:96. Nina Carlier, Victoria S. Marshe, Jana Cmorejova, Caroline Davis, and Daniel J. Müller, "Genetic Similarities between Compulsive Overeating and Addiction Phenotypes: A Case

for 'Food Addiction'?" *Current Psychiatry Reports*: December 2015, 17 (12): 96.

17) Caroline Davis et al., "Evidence that 'food addiction' is a valid phenotype of obesity," *Appetite* 57, no. 3 (2011): 711–17.

18) See NEDA: Feeding Hope. Statistics and Research on Eating Disorders. https://www.nationaleatingdisorders.org/statistics-research-eating-disorders

CHAPTER FIVE
ARE YOU A FOOD ADDICT?

1) These are a few of the twenty questions that many of the food twelve-step groups use to determine if someone is a food addict. For the full twenty questions, see *www.foodaddicts.org*.

2) To access these three thousand peer-reviewed writings, see www.food addictioninstitute.org/FAI-DOCS/Full-Bibliography.pdf.

3) See Michael Moss, *Salt Sugar Fat: How the Food Giants Hooked Us* (New York: Random House, 2013) for an excellent treatise on the subject.

4) Both Drs. Frank Minirth and Paul Meier oversee clinics that provide Christian-based behavioural health services, including treatments for addiction, anxiety, depression, grief, and PTSD. See www.theminirth clinic.com and www.meierclinics.com.

5) Published in 1985, Judi Hollis's *Fat Is a Family Affair* (Center City, MN: Hazelden Foundation) was required reading for most patients admitted for treatment of food addiction at rehabilitation centres during the eighties and nineties. The book's original subtitle was *A Guide for People with Eating Disorders and Those Who Love Them*. Later editions changed the subtitle to *How Food Obsessions Affect Relationships*. The text is widely recognized as the benchmark reference on family dynamics and eating disorders.

6) William Rader founded The Rader Institute in 1984. Not focused on weight loss, it was specifically tailored for patients suffering from anorexia, bulimia, and compulsive overeating.

7) As head of the U.S. National Institute on Drug Abuse, Dr. Nora D. Volkow is an influential figure and her statements carry extra weight.

Her focus on addiction of *all* types as a brain disease has been widely heralded. See Nora D. Vokow and R.A. Wise, "How can drug addiction help us understand obesity?" *Nature Neuroscience* 8, no. 5 (2005): 555–60.

8) The American Society of Addiction Medicine has proposed their own set of criteria to capture the larger scope of addictions that have been recognized since the *DSM-IV* (Diagnostic and Statistics Manual) was introduced. These are the ABCDEs of addiction. These, too, are applicable to many of us who struggle with food addiction:

- Abstinence: Once attempted, is the person able to become abstinent?
- Behavioural Control: Is the person able to control their behaviour around their drug intake?
- Cravings: Does the person crave or obsess about their drug of choice?
- Diminishment of Consequences/Denial: Does the person lack insight into how problematic his drug use is?
- Emotional Regulation: Is the person emotionally volatile? Does the person have an abnormal emotional relationship to his drug of choice?

9) For those of us working in the field of food addiction, the *DSM-IV* (Diagnostic and Statistics Manual) has been a poor reflection of our clinical reality. The highly controversial *DSM-5*, released in May 2013, is not much of an improvement over the *DSM-IV* for the food addict. Those working in the eating disorders field have achieved landmark success in getting binge eating disorder (BED) recognized as a clinical entity that exists apart from anorexia and bulimia. This diagnosis now includes persons who suffer from the uncontrollable urge to eat large amounts of food (usually in intermittent sessions). Thus, many of those who are obese can now get fundable treatment, outside of bariatric surgery.

The lack of a diagnosis of food addiction in the *DSM,* however, means that nothing much has changed for food addicts. Many are now diagnosed as suffering from binge eating disorder, and if they are given treatment for that disorder, the treatment could ultimately undermine their recovery. Modified diets do not work for the food addict.

10) See Ashley Gerhardt et al., "Yale Food Addiction Scale," www.yale ruddcenter.org/resources/upload/docs/what/addiction/FoodAddic tionScale09.pdf. For a discussion of early results, see also Ashley Gearhardt et al., "Preliminary Validation of the Yale Food Addiction Scale," *Appetite* 52 (2008): 430–36.

11) Developed in 2009 and studied for its effectiveness in 2014, the Yale Food Addiction Scale (YFAS) remains the only scientifically respected and validated measure of addictive-like eating behaviour. In its original form, the scale was tailored to reflect the *DSM-IV-TR* criteria for addiction. When those criteria were changed for the *DSM-5*, the YFAS was also updated to mirror the new diagnostic profile.

A subsequent study by Gearhardt, et al., published in 2016, reported that the newer YFAS is a valid tool for self-reported measurements of disordered eating. Their research indicates that the updated version's findings are consistent with those recorded using the initial YFAS.

CHAPTER SIX
THE FOOD FIGHTS: ADDICTION OR EATING DISORDER?

1) See Frank M. Sacks et al., "Comparison of Weight Loss Diets with Different Compositions of Fat, Protein, and Carbohydrates," *New England Journal of Medicine* 360, no. 9 (2009): 859–73 for a good example of a work that prompts the conclusion that "calorie intake alone determines how successful a diet will be."

2) As an example of how professionals tended to view eating disorders, see Christopher Fairburn and G. Terrence Wilson, *Binge Eating Disorder: Nature, Assessment and Treatment* (New York: Guilford Press, 1996). Subsequent works by the authors leaned more toward self-help diet books. In 2013, Fairburn penned *Overcoming Binge Eating, Second Edition: The Proven Program to Learn Why You Binge and How You Can Stop* (New York: Guilford Press), and in 2007 Wilson co-authored with Janet D. Latner *Self-Help Approaches for Obesity and Eating Disorders: Research and Practice* (New York: Guilford Press, 2007).

3) Sheppard, Katherine, and Ifland are all self-proclaimed food addicts themselves. Their books are prescribed and read widely by recovering food addicts and those with eating disorders. Sheppard is author of *Food Addiction: The Body Knows* (Deerfield Beach, FL: Health Communications, 1993), Katherine wrote *Anatomy of a Food Addiction: The Brain Chemistry of Overeating* (Carlsbad, CA: Gurze Books, 1996) and Ifland offered *Sugars and Flours: How They Make Us Crazy, Sick, and Fat and What to Do about It* (Bloomington, IL: AuthorHouse, 2000). In 2008, Ifland also collaborated on a paper titled "Refined food addiction: A classic substance use disorder," which is available on Elsevier's website (www.elsevier.com).

4) Organized in 1985, the International Association of Eating Disorder Professionals touts its annual symposium as an event that "draws attendees from all corners of the globe, including especially numerous professionals from the United States, Canada, Mexico, Brazil and the United Kingdom." There is little discussion about addiction. For an illustration, see "iaedp Symposium 2012," www. regonline.com/builder/site/tab2.aspx?EventID=984977.

5) Although the Overeaters Anonymous fellowship's members remain anonymous, the OA World Service Office has collected valuable data from its members. See "2010 Membership Survey Report," *Overeaters Anonymous, www.oa.org/ pdfs/2010_Member_Survey.pdf.*

6) Carin Gorrell, "Sarah Ferguson: The Duchess Weighs In," Psychology Today, January 1, 2002. Last reviewed June 9, 2016. https://www. psychologytoday.com/ca/articles/200201/sarah-ferguson-the-duchess -weighs-in?collection=10061.

7) "Lose weight your way: 9,000 readers rate 13 diet plans and tools," *Consumer Reports* (February 2013): 26–28, summarizes the magazine's most recent research. Researchers James Hill and Rena Wing peg the number of successful weight losers at closer to 20 percent. See their discussion in "The National Weight Control Registry," *The Permanente Jou*rnal 7, no. 3 (Summer 2003): 1–73.

8) K.A. Gudzune, R.S. Doshi, A.K. Mehta, Z.W. Chaudhry, D.K. Jacobs, R.M.Vakil, C.J. Lee, S.N. Bleich, J.M. Clark, "Efficacy of commercial weight-loss programs: an updated systematic review,"

Annals of Internal Medicine 8 (April 7 2015): 501–12, doi: 10.7326/
M14-2238.

9) Anorexic actor Portia de Rossi authored a popular memoir titled
Unbearable Lightness: A Story of Loss and Gain (New York: Atria
Books, 2011). Olympic gymnast Cathy Rigby began talking publicly
about her bulimia and anorexia in the eighties. She was interviewed
for an article in C. McCoy (Rigby), "A Onetime Olympic Gymnast
Overcomes the Bulimia That Threatened Her Life," *People* (August 13,
1984): 68–72. While Princess Diana's bulimia was widely discussed
in the press, a good source of her own thoughts about her illness is
Andrew Morton, *Diana: Her True Story in Her Own Words* (New York:
Simon & Schuster, 1997).

10) See "Eating Disorder Statistics," *Mirror Mirror*, www.mirror-mirror.
org/eating-disorders-statistics.htm.

11) Fotios C. Papadopoulos et al., "Excess mortality causes of death and
prognostic factors in anorexia nervosa," *British Journal of Psychiatry*
194 (2009): 10–17.

CHAPTER EIGHT
STAGES OF FOOD ADDICTION

1) The stages of addiction — early stage, middle stage, late stage, final
stage — were first conceptualized with the use of the Jellinek Curve,
named for E. Morton Jellinek, author of *The Disease Concept of
Alcoholism* (New Haven, CT: Hillhouse, 1960). Phil Werdell has utilized this paradigm with food addiction, based on his extensive clinical exposure to food addicts through ACORN Food Dependency
Recovery Services.

2) Angry voices in the nutritional community claim that we are actually
committing pediacide by allowing our children to eat sugary foods
such as breakfast cereals, soda pop, and pizza lunches. Even the fruit
juices proposed for healthy school lunch programs are loaded with
sugar and other unhealthy ingredients. Advocates of healthy eating
recommend that we ban these foods, especially from school cafeterias;
others say that we should go further and tax junk food. Some even
advocate such harsh measures such as removing obese children from

the homes of their parents. They state that to encourage children to eat these foods in the name of convenience or cheaper cost is tantamount to child abuse. See Robert H. Lustig, *Fat Chance: Beating the Odds Against Sugar, Processed Food, Obesity, and Disease* (New York: Penguin Plume, 2012) for more discussion of these proposals.

3) Research on the effectiveness of weight-loss or bariatric surgery has been going on since the first attempt at this treatment, conducted in 1954. It wasn't until 1967, however, that surgeon Edward E. Mason at the University of Iowa developed the first gastric bypass surgery (referred to as intestinal bypass at the time) after noticing that people who had large portions of their stomachs or intestines surgically removed because of surgery for cancer or ulcers had dramatic weight loss no matter how much they ate. For a discussion of considerations before weight-loss surgery, see Philip Werdell, *Bariatric Surgery & Food Addiction: Pre-operative Considerations* (Sarasota, FL: EverGreen Publications, 2009).

CHAPTER NINE
FOOD ADDICTION: THE GREAT SABOTEUR

1) As the former president of the Corn Refiners Association, Audrae Erickson comments most often in defense of high fructose corn syrup as a benign sweetener. She issued a public statement in 2006, however, which said, in part, "it is important to note that many factors contribute to the development of obesity."

2) For detailed suggestions for losing weight, see www.livestrong.com/weight-loss/. See also, www.loseit.com. This entire website is dedicated to helping the dieter track calories and exercise, and find support through social media.

3) See Adrian Meule, "How Prevalent is 'Food Addiction'?" *Frontiers in Psychiatry* 2, no. 61 (2011).

4) See Ashley Gearhardt et al., "Yale Food Addiction Scale," www.yale ruddcenter.org/resources/upload/docs/what/addiction/FoodAddic tionScale09.pdf. For a discussion of early results, see also Ashley Gearhardt et al., "Preliminary Validation of the Yale Food Addiction Scale," *Appetite* 52 (2008): 430–36.

5) We learn the fascinating story of fitness guru Jack LaLanne at www. biography.com/people/jack-lalanne-273648. According to The Biography Channel, "As a child, he ate a lot of sugary foods and got into trouble at school. 'I was a sugarholic and a junk food junkie! It made me weak and it made me mean,' LaLanne said. But he completely changed his life around after attending a lecture by a nutritionist as a teenager. LaLanne cut out sugar and other unhealthy foods from his diet and began exercising."

6) No longer offering treatment for food addiction, Glenbeigh of Tampa is a psychiatric hospital that offered a highly successful twelve-step based program from 1986 until the mid-1990s. Patients stayed at the residential facility for four to six weeks, were given a specific no-sugar/no-flour food plan, participated in daily process groups, were encouraged to meditate and exercise, and attended lectures on the nature of addiction.

7) The first ACORN survey was conducted in 2006. It was repeated in subsequent years. See Philip Werdell, *Food Addiction Recovery, A New Model of Professional Support: The ACORN Primary Intensive* (Sarasota, FL: EverGreen Publications, 2007). M.T. Carroll surveyed alumni and alumnae of the Glenbeigh food addiction treatment program and found that 90 percent were able to achieve abstinence. One-third were able to maintain abstinence for one to five years, one-third had a slip or break but recovered their abstinence, and one-third were unable to stay abstinent. See M.T. Carroll, "The Eating Disorder Inventory and Other Predictors of Successful Symptom Management of Bulimic and Obese Women Following an Inpatient Treatment Program Employing the Addictive Paradigm," Ph.D. diss.(University of South Florida, 1993).

CHAPTER TEN
FOR THE ANOREXIC

1) For an overview of jockeys and eating disorders, see "A Jockey's Hard Life," PBS.org, www.pbs.org/wgbh/americanexperience/features/general-article/seabiscuit-jockeys-hard-life/, and Mark Hughes, "Jockeys 'run risk of eating disorders' in bid to stay slim," *Independent*,

last updated March 11, 2008, www.independent.co.uk/sport/racing/jockeys-run-risk-of-eating-disorders-in-bid-to-stay-slim-793964.html.

2) For more information about Renae Norton's clinic, services, and her survey of bulimorexia, see her website, www.eatingdisorderpro.com/home/.

3) Success rates with eating disorders is, at best, 60 percent. Most clinicians agree that intensive inpatient treatment is required to achieve long-term success. Unfortunately, it has been estimated that only one in ten individuals will seek treatment for their eating disorder.

   In a ten-year review of eating disorders treatment, McAleavey (2008) estimates that the long-term success rate (beyond five years) of recovery from eating disorder behaviours is actually only 40 to 50 percent, and much lower if using randomized controlled trials to test the efficacy of treatment. This researcher attributes the poverty of success to the "failure to appreciate that BN and BED have addiction components that might require twelve-step or multimodal approaches."

CHAPTER ELEVEN
HITTING BOTTOM: I NEED HELP!

1) Adelle Davis was one of the country's best-known nutritionists and often considered the mother of the health food movement. She authored four bestsellers: *Let's Cook It Right*, *Let's Have Healthy Children*, *Let's Get Well*, and *Let's Eat Right To Keep Fit*. This last book, first published in 1954, became the bible to the many overweight people who turned to natural and organic food plans as a weight loss strategy. See www.adelledavis.org/adelle-davis/.

2) Phil Werdell has held teaching and/or professorship positions at Yale University, City University of New York, Kansas State University, and the University of New Hampshire.

CHAPTER TWELVE
WHAT DO I DO NOW?

1) See Anemona Hartocollis, "Young, Obese and In Surgery," *New York Times* (January 8, 2012): A1. The author also states that this number

of 220,000 bypass surgeries is a "sevenfold leap in a decade, according to industry figures — costing more than $6 billion a year."

2) Dr. Yoni Feedhoff, founder of the Ottawa Bariatric Medical Institute, commented on a report about bariatric surgeries that was released in May 2014 by the Canadian Institute for Health Information. It covers the seven-year period from 2006–2007 to 2012–2013. The report only captures surgeries performed by provincial health-care programs. Gastric bypass surgeries that were paid for by individuals or which were done outside of Canada are not included. See Helen Branswell, "Bariatric Surgery Numbers Up Significantly in Canada but Annual Figures Still Low," CTV News, last modified May 22, 2014, www. ctvnews.ca/health/bariatric-surgery-numbers-up-significantly-in-canada-but-annual-figures-still-low-1.1833663.

3) Adams, T., Davidson L., et al. "Weight and Metabolic Outcomes 12 Years after Gastric Bypass", *New England Journal of Medicine*, 377 (2017): 1143–55.

4) Here is an example of specific instructions given to patients after bar-iatric surgery. AVOID:
   - Sugar and sugary foods, including high-calorie soft drinks, syrups, honey, jelly, jam, cakes, cookies, candy, ice cream.
   - High-fat foods, including chocolate, chips, pies, pastries, ice cream, bacon, sausage, fried foods, cream soups, cream sauces.
   - High-calorie drinks, such as milkshakes, soda, beer, orange juice, apple juice, other fruit juices, whole milk.
   - Starchy and white-flour foods, such as pasta, rice, and doughy breads.
   - Fats such as butter or oil should be restricted to three to four teaspoons per day.

5) See Philip Werdell, "Overview of Bariatric Surgery," *Bariatric Surgery & Food Addiction: Preoperative Considerations* (Sarasota, FL: EverGreen Publications, 2009) and the National Association for Weight Loss Surgery (www.nawls. com).

6) The American Society for Bariatric Surgery has adopted strict guide-lines for bypass eligibility. To be a good candidate for weight loss

surgery, patients must have had a body mass index above forty (morbidly obese) for at least five years or a BMI more than 35 (obese) along with an obesity-related medical problem such as Type 2 diabetes. They must be between the ages of eighteen and sixty-five, although that seems to be changing as more adolescents are being approved for weight loss operations on a case-by-case basis.

Patients must also pass a psychological screening test to weed out anyone suffering from mental illness. Some insurance companies insist that patients prove they have tried to lose weight through a medically supervised program before seeking surgery. See "Information on Bariatric Surgery," *U.S. News & World Report*, last modified January 2010, www.health.usnews.com.

7) For more information about the higher risk of alcohol abuse after bariatric surgery, see W.C. King et al., "Prevalence of Alcohol Use Disorders Before and After Bariatric Surgery," *Journal of the American Medical Association* 307 (2012): 2516–25. See also Smith K.E. et al. "Problematic Alcohol Use and Associated Characteristics Following Bariatric Surgery," *Obesity Surgery*. 2017.

8) See "Weight Loss Surgery Increases Risk of Alcohol Addiction," *ABC News, Good Morning, America,* last modified June 2012, www.abc news.go.com/Health/Wellness.

9) The figure of $40 billion spent on the American diet industry was reported in 2005 by BankRate.com, where the total was projected to rise to $48 billion by 2006. PRWeb.com reported that revenues for the total U.S. weight loss market were actually *$60.9 billion* in 2010, and $60.4 billion in 2009.

10) These estimates come from "Forget Diet Pills, Try Oatmeal," an *ABC News* feature broadcast in October 2005 and repeated on *Good Morning America* in December 2005.

11) See Elizabeth Bernstein, "A New Breed of 'Diet' Pills," *The Wall Street Journal,* August 22, 2006; and Tracii Hanes, "Zoloft & Weight Gain or Loss," LIVESTRONG, last modified September 2010, www. livestrong.org; and Karen Frazier, "How Does Topamax Help Weight Loss?" LIVESTRONG, last modified June 2011, www. live strong.org.

12) For more information on Qsymia and Belviq, see John M. Grohol, "Qsymia and Belviq Drugs for Obesity, Weight Loss," *Pscyh Central*, last modified 2012, www. psychcentral.com, and "Medications Target Long-Term Weight Control," *U.S. Food and Drug Administration*, last modified July 2012, www.fda.gov.

13) See "FDA Announces Withdrawal of Fenfluramine and Dexfen-fluramine (Fen-Phen)," *U.S. Food and Drug Administration*, last modified September 1997, www. fda.gov/Drugs/DrugSafety.

14) For a brief explanation, see also "Contingency Management Interventions/Motivational Incentives," *U.S. National Institute on Drug Abuse*, last modified December 2012, www.drugabuse.gov/publi cations. For a current list of UCHC contingency management research papers, see www.contingencymanagement. uchc.edu/trials_projects.

   There are also dozens of studies on the effectiveness of various psychotherapies utilized with bulimics and those with binge eating disorder. See David Garner et al., "A comparison of cognitive-behavioral and supportive-expressive therapy for bulimia nervosa," *American Journal of Psychiatry* 150, no. 1 (1993): 37–46l and P.J. Hay et al., "Psychotherapy for bulimia nervosa and bingeing," *Cochrane Database of Systematic Reviews* 3 (2003): 1–73.

CHAPTER THIRTEEN
FIRST THINGS FIRST: STOPPING THE FOOD

1) When grains are refined, the sugar they contain becomes more accessible, easier and faster to digest. As a result, the effects for the food and/or sugar addict are much the same as those experienced from eating sugar itself. Refined flour (especially that from wheat) has also been linked to loss of control, a problem related to the substance's gluten content. Gluten activates celiac disease and gluten intolerance. See Joan Ifland, *Sugars and Flours: How They Make Us Crazy, Sick and Fat and What to Do About It* (Bloomington, IL: AuthorHouse, 2003) and www.celiac.org. See also Mark Cheren, "Physical craving and food addiction: a review of the science," *Food Addiction Institute*, www.foodaddictioninstitute.org.

2) See William Davis, *Wheat Belly: Lose the Wheat, Lose the Weight, and Find Your Way Back to Health* (New York: HarperCollins, 2012). Although Davis acknowledges the addictive nature of foods, particularly wheat (using the glycemic index) and sugar, this book is primarily focused on the health consequences of wheat. Davis coined a useful phase: "'Bread is Solid Beer' and 'Beer is Liquid Bread.'" What is the difference between the two? Yeast and time of fermentation. Not even yeast, it turns out — you can make alcohol out of yeast designated for bread making. This may be why alcoholics hate to give up their sugar *as well as* their bread. Davis explores the neurochemistry to show how the differences between the two are not so stark.

3) Two papers presented by Sarah H. Leibowitz at the annual Obesity and Food Addiction Summit, "Mechanisms of Food Cravings," (2009) and "Overconsumption of Fats: A Vicious Cycle from the Start" (2007), look at the addictive potential of fat alone.

4) See M. Yanina Pepino et al., "Sucralose Affects Glycemic and Hormonal Responses to an Oral Glucose Load," *Diabetes Care* 36, no. 9 (September 2013): 2530–35. To the human brain, sweet is sweet. A study of bulimics and anorexics found they were just as likely to binge on artificial sugar as they were on real sugar. See D.A. Klein et al., "Artificial sweetener use among individuals with eating disorders," *International Journal of Eating Disorders* 39, no. 4 (2006): 341–45. In fact, it has been shown that rats prefer artificially sweetened food over cocaine. See Magalie Lenoir et al., "Intense Sweetness Surpasses Cocaine Reward," *PLoS ONE* 2, no. 8 (2007): 698. See also Pepino et al. "Sucralose Affects Glycemic and Hormonal Responses to an Oral Glucose Load," *Diabetes Care* (Sep 2013) 2530-5, and Azad et al., "Nonnutritive sweeteners and cardiometabolic health: a systematic review and meta-analysis of randomized controlled trials and prospective cohort studies", *CMAJ* (July 17, 2017) E929–E939.

5) Food addicts who are sensitive to sugar have learned to look for it in ingredient lists under multiple names. *Prevention* provides a list of the most popular terms. These include evaporated cane juice, high fructose corn syrup, agave, as well as some of the more esoteric (barley malt, golden syrup, diastatic malt, diastase, treacle, panocha, sorghum

syrup). See "10 Sneaky Names for Sugar" at www. prevention.com, and "Names of Sugar" at www.foodaddictsanonymous.org.

6) The official explanation for the glycemic index comes from the Human Nutrition Unit, School of Molecular Biosciences, University of Sydney, Australia: "The glycemic index (GI) is a ranking of carbohydrates on a scale from 0 to 100 according to the extent to which they raise blood sugar levels after eating." See www. glycemicindex.com.

7) Each food addict determines what her individual trigger foods are. Typically these include sweets (candy, ice cream, pie, cake, cupcakes, cookies, donuts, etc.), flour products (bread, bagels, pasta, rolls, pizza, etc.), and crunchy snacks (potato chips, corn chips, nuts, pretzels, popcorn, etc.). Less often they include meat, butter, high-fat dairy products (cheese, cream cheese, sour cream, whole milk, etc.), and fried foods (chicken and chicken "nuggets," french fries, fish sticks, etc.).

Food behaviours can also be triggers; these usually relate to overeating in quantities, hoarding food, scarfing food, gulping food, regurgitating food, stealing food, and restricting food.

8) See Gabor Maté, *In the Realm of the Hungry Ghosts: Close Encounters with Addiction* (Berkeley, CA: North Atlantic Books, 2010) for an excellent discussion of addiction to drugs and alcohol.

9) There are a number of programs that are now claiming to treat food addiction, but few are appropriate for a bona fide food addict. Here are some questions to ask when evaluating a program that claims to treat food addiction:

- What type of food plan does the program advocate? Is it free of sugar, flour, excess fat, alcohol, caffeine?
- Does the program measure the success rate of its graduates? What percentage of graduates have managed continuous abstinence for a year or more after treatment?

10) For more information on ACORN Food Dependency Recovery Services, see http://foodaddiction.com.

11) Theresa Wright, MS, RD, LDN, founded Renaissance Nutrition Center, Inc. in 1990 in East Norriton, Pennsylvania. She creates and teaches nutrition and weight management programs, and, after thirty-five years in various health-care roles, now focuses her extensive practice

on the treatment of addictive and compulsive eating disorders. See www.sanefood.com.

12) M.T. Carroll surveyed alumni and alumnae of the Glenbeigh food addiction treatment program and found that 90 percent were able to achieve abstinence. One-third were able to maintain abstinence for one to five years, one-third had a slip or break but recovered their abstinence, and one-third were unable to stay abstinent. See M.T. Carroll, "The Eating Disorder Inventory and Other Predictors of Successful Symptom Management of Bulimic and Obese Women Following an Inpatient Treatment Program Employing the Addictive Paradigm," Ph.D. diss. (University of South Florida, 1993).

13) According to Harm Reduction International (formerly the International Harm Reduction Association), "harm reduction refers to policies, programs and practices that aim to reduce the harms associated with the use of psychoactive drugs in people unable or unwilling to stop." With regard to food addiction, this translates into fewer relapses, binges, or purges rather than complete abstinence from those episodes. See www.ihra.net.

14) Here are some excellent meal plans for a non-food addict. Most come from the "paleo" community. Food addicts can also benefit once they have identified and eliminated their trigger foods, which may still be offered in these meal plans:
   - www.dietdoctor.com/lchf
   - http://robbwolf.com/what-is-the-paleo-diet/meal-plans-shopping-guides/
   - http://cavemanstrong.com/food/meal-plans/
   - www.deliverlean.com/paleo-diet-plan.aspx
   - http://paleodietlifestyle.com/paleo-meal-plan/
   - www.livestrong.com/article/222874-paleo-diet-meal-plans/
   - www.multiplydelicious.com/thefood/2012/01/weekly-paleo-meal-plan/
   - http://primaltoad.com/day1/
   - www.elanaspantry.com/paleo-diet-recipes/
   - http://home.trainingpeaks.com/articles/nutrition/quick-guide- the-paleo-diet-for-athletes.aspx

- http://unitedbarbell.com/dox/30%20Day%20Paleo%20 Challenge%20Packet.pdf
- www.foodonthetable.com/content/paleo-diet-meal-plan/
- www.primalpal.net/home
- www.paleoplan.com/resources/sampler-menu-meal-plan/
- www.thepaleodietmealplan.com/paleo-diet-blog/
- www.paleoplan.com/resources/sampler-menu-meal-plan/

15) Here are some resources that have been proven to work specifically for food addicts. We have also included some specific food plans that you may wish to consider.
   - www.foodaddictsanonymous.org/faa-food-plan
   - www.foodaddiction.com/Publications/Food%20Plan%20 As%20 a%20Tool.html
   - http://recovery.hiwaay.net/foodplans/how.html

16) Clinicians sometimes eschew structured food plans as being "too rigid," for fear they will lead to anorexia or, at minimum, unbearable feelings of deprivation. Melinda Johnson, "The Diet Mentality Paradox: Why Dieting Can Make You Fat," *U.S. News & World Report*, last modified August 17, 2012, http://health.usnews.com/ health-news/blogs/eat-run/2012/08/17/the-diet-mentality-paradox-why-dieting-can-make-you-fat. See also T.M. Stewart et al., "Rigid vs. flexible dieting: association with eating disorder symptoms in non-obese women," *Appetite* 38, no. 1 (2002): 39–44.

CHAPTER FIFTEEN
SWITCHING ADDICTIONS

1) See "The Family Afterward" in *Alcoholics Anonymous* (New York: Alcoholics Anonymous World Services, 2001). This chapter notes twice that eating sweets — at least in 1939 — was an acceptable and *recommended* way to stave off a craving for alcohol.

CHAPTER SIXTEEN
FREEDOM TASTES GREAT! FINDING FOOD SERENITY

1) The Founders of Alcoholics Anonymous were Bill Wilson and Dr. Bob Smith. Bill Wilson was a stockbroker and the primary author of

the AA text, *Alcoholics Anonymous.* Bob Smith was a doctor who got sober after meeting with Bill on May 12, 1935. The fellowship officially began in 1939, with the publication of their primer, *Alcoholics Anonymous.* An excellent source for understanding the roots of the twelve-step program can be found in Ernest Kurtz's *Not-God: A History of Alcoholics Anonymous* (Center City, MN: Hazelden Educational Materials, 1979). See also www.aa.org/aatimeline/.

2) In 1985, the National Institutes of Health Consensus Development Conference on the Health Implications of Obesity defined the obesity as a BMI (body mass index) of 27.8 for men and 27.3 for women. See B.T. Burton and W.R. Foster, "Health implications of obesity: NIH Consensus Development Conference," *International Journal of Obesity* 9, no. 3 (1986): 155–70.

Before this, in 1942, the first edition of the Metropolitan Life Insurance Company listed weight and height tables outlining ideal weight ranges; individuals outside of range were considered overweight or underweight. See www.halls.md/ideal-weight/met.htm.

3) As noted, there are nine different fellowships for food addicts. The list of food-related twelve-step groups includes: Overeaters Anonymous (OA), Overeaters Anonymous-HOW (OA-HOW), 90-Day OA (OA 90 Day), Food Addicts Anonymous (FAA), Food Addicts in Recovery Anonymous (FA), Compulsive Eaters Anonymous HOW (CEA-HOW), GreySheeters Anonymous (GSA), Eating Disorders Anonymous (EDA), and Recovering Food Addicts Anonymous (RFA). The Christian fellowship Overcomers Anonymous (Overcomers) is for all addictions, including compulsive eating and food addiction.

4) See Imke Janssen et al., "Testosterone and Visceral Fat in Midlife Women: The Study of Women's Health Across the Nation (SWAN) Fat Patterning Study," *Obesity* 18, no. 3 (March 2010): 604–10.

5) See Lyn-Genet Recitas, *The Plan: Eliminate the Surprising "Healthy" Foods That Are Making You Fat — and Lose Weight Fast* (London: Orion, 2013).

EPILOGUE: A HAPPY ENDING, ONE DAY AT A TIME

1) This is a reference both to the Tibetan analogy of addiction, and, of course, to Gabor Maté's book on addiction, *In the Realm of Hungry Ghosts* (Berkeley, CA: North Atlantic Books, 2010). This is an excellent description of addiction, based on science, personal experience, as well as the experiences of hard-core heroin addicts from the downtown east side of Vancouver.

BIBLIOGRAPHY

Adamo, Ann. "U.S. Weight Loss and Diet Trends 2016-2017." Accessed October 28, 2016. Women's Marketing. http://www.womensmarketing.com/blog/u.s.-weight-loss-and-diet-trends-2016-wmi.

Adams, Kelly M., Martin Kohlmeier, and Steven H. Zeisel. "Nutrition Education in U.S. Medical Schools: Latest Update of a National Survey." *Journal of the Association of American Medical College* 85, no. 9 (2010): 1537–42.

Adams, T., Davidson L, et al. "Weight and Metabolic Outcomes 12 Years after Gastric Bypass," *New England Journal of Medicine* 377 (2017): 1143–55.

Alcoholics Anonymous. New York: Alcoholics Anonymous World Services, 2001. American Psychiatric Association. *Diagnostic and Statistical Manual of Mental Disorders.* 4th ed. Arlington, VA: American Psychiatric Publishing, 2000.

American Psychological Association. "The Impact of Food Advertising on Childhood Obesity." American Psychological Association. www.apa.org/topics/kids-media/food.aspx.

Andrews, R.A. "Patient information: Weight loss surgery (Beyond the Basics)." Up To Date. Last modified March 20, 2013. www.uptodate.com/contents weight-loss-surgery-beyond-the-basics?source=search_result&search=bariatric+surgery&selectedTitle=8%7E95.

Avena, Nicole M. "Sugar-dependent rats show enhanced intake of unsweetened ethanol." *Alcohol* 34 (2004): 203–09.

Avena, Nicole M., and Bartley G. Hoebel. "A diet promoting sugar dependency causes behavioral cross-sensitization to a low dose of amphetamine." *Neuroscience* 122, no. 1 (2003): 17–20.

Avena, Nicole M., and John R. Talbott. *Why Diets Fail (Because You're Addicted to Sugar): Science Explains How to End Cravings, Lose Weight, and Get Healthy.* New York: Ten Speed Press, 2014.

Avena, Nicole M., Pedro Rada, and Bartley G. Hoebel. "Evidence for sugar addiction: Behavioral and neurochemical effects of intermittent, excessive sugar intake." *Neuroscience and Biobehavioral Reviews* 32, no. 1 (2008): 20–39.

Avena, Nicole M. *Hedonic Eating: How the Pleasure of Food Affects our Brains and Behaviour.* Oxford University Press, 2015.

Barry, Danielle, Megan Clarke, and Nancy M. Petry. "Obesity and Its Relationship to Addictions: Is Overeating a Form of Addictive Behavior?" *American Journal on Addictions* 18 (2009): 439–51.

Bernstein, Elizabeth. "A New Breed of 'Diet' Pills." *Wall Street Journal,* August 22, 2006.

"Best Diet Rankings." U.S. News & World Report. http://health.usnews.com/best-diet/best-weight-loss-diets?int=ea2125.

Blumentahl, D.M., and M.S. Gold. "Neurobiology of food addiction." *Current Opinion in Clinical Nutrition and Metabolic Care* 13 (2010): 359–65.

Bocarsly, Miriam E., et al. "Rats that binge eat fat-rich food do not show somatic signs or anxiety associated with opiate-like withdrawal: implications for nutrient-specific food addiction behaviors." *Physiology & Behavior* 104, no. 5 (2011): 865–72.

Bozarth, Michael A. "Pleasure Systems in the Brain." In *Pleasure: The Politics and the Reality,* edited by D.M. Warburton. New York: John Wiley & Sons, 1994.

Branswell, Helen. "Bariatric Surgery Numbers Up Significantly in Canada but Annual Figures Still Low." CTV News. Last modified May 22, 2014. www.ctvnews.ca/health/bariatric-surgery-numbers-up-significantly-in-canada-but-annual-figures-still-low-1.1833663.

Breuning, Loretta. *Meet Your Happy Chemicals.* Pomona, CA: System Integrity Press, 2012.

Brewerton, Timothy and Amy Dennis, eds. *Eating Disorders, Addictions and Substance Use Disorders: Research, Clinical and Treatment Perspectives.* Berlin: Springer Science and Business Media, 2014.

Brown, Harriet. "The Weight of the Evidence." Slate. Accessed March 24, 2015. http://www.slate.com/articles/health_and_science/medical_examiner/2015/03/diets_do_not_work_the_thin_evidence_that_losing_weight_makes_you_healthier.html.

Brownell, Kelly D. "Thinking Forward: The Quicksand of Appeasing the Food Industry." *PLoS Medicine* 9, no. 7 (2012): 1–2.

Burrows, Tracey, et al. "Food Addiction, Binge Eating Disorder and Obesity: Is There a Relationship?" *Behavioral Sciences* 7 no. 3 (2017): E54. https://dx.doi.org/10.3390%2Fbs7030054.

Burton, B.T., and W.R. Foster. "Health implications of obesity: NIH Consensus Development Conference." *International Journal of Obesity* 9, no. 3 (1986): 155–70.

Canadian Obesity Network, 2017. *Report Card on Access to Obesity Treatment for Adults in Canada,* 2017.

Carlier, N., et al. "Genetic Similarities between Compulsive Overeating and Addiction Phenotypes: A Case for "Food Addiction." *Current Psychiatry Reports* 17 no. 12 (2015): 96.

Carroll, Mary Theodora. "The Eating Disorder Inventory and Other Predictors of Successful Symptom Management of Bulimic and Obese Women Following an Inpatient Treatment Program Employing the Addictive Paradigm." Ph.D. diss., University of South Florida, 1993.

Clayton, Christine. "State Laws Aimed at Improving School Meals Help Teens Eat More Fruits and Vegetables, New Study Finds." Press release from Robert Wood Johnson Foundation, based on research published in *American Journal of Preventive Medicine,* March 12, 2013.

Collins, Judy. Cravings: *How I Conquered Food: A Memoir.* Nan. A. Talese, 2017.

"Compass of Pleasure: Why Some Things Feel So Good." *Fresh Air.* National Public Radio, June 23, 2001.

"Cupcakes may be addictive, just like cocaine." Langreth, R., and Standord D., Nov 2, 2011. Bloomberg. https://www.bloomberg.com/news/articles/2011-11-02/fatty-foods-addictive-as-cocaine-in-growing-body-of-science.

Dallman, Mary F. "Stress-induced obesity and the emotional nervous system." *Trends in Endocrinology and Metabolism* 21, no. 3 (2010): 159–65.

Davidson, Steven. "Understanding and Treating Cross Addictions." Paper presented at the 7th Annual Tennessee Drug Court Conference, 2010.

Davis, Caroline, et al. "Dopamine for 'Wanting' and Opioids for 'Liking': A Comparison of Obese Adults With and Without Binge Eating." *Obesity* 17 (2009): 1220–25.

———. "Evidence that 'food addiction' is a valid phenotype of obesity." *Appetite* 57, no. 3 (2011): 711–17.

Davis, William. *Wheat Belly: Lose the Wheat, Lose the Weight, and Find Your Way Back to Health.* New York: Harper Collins Publishers, 2012.

Dayton, Tian. "Are You Self-Medicating Your Emotional Stress with Food?" *Huffington Post.* Last modified February 25, 2010. www.huffington post.com/dr-tian-dayton/are- you-self-medicating-y_b_476399.html.

de Rossi, Portia. *Unbearable Lightness: A Story of Loss and Gain.* New York: Atria Books, 2011.

di Chiara, Gaetano, and Assunta Imperato. "Drugs abused by humans preferentially increase synaptic dopamine concentrations in the mesolimbic system of freely moving rats." *Proceedings of the National Academy of Sciences of the United States of America* 85, no. 14 (July 1988): 5274–78.

Drewnowski, Adam, et al. "Naloxone, an opiate blocker, reduces the consumption of sweet high-fat foods in obese and lean female binge eaters." *American Journal of Clinical Nutrition* 61, no. 6 (1995): 1206–12.

Dufty, William. *Sugar Blues.* Radnor, PA: Chilton Book Company, 1975.

Dworkin-McDaniel, Norine. "Are You a Food Addict?" *More* (September 2012): 152–58.

Edwards, C. "The Sugar Racket." *Cato Institute Tax & Budget Bulletin* 4 (June 2007): 1–2.

Epstein, David, and Yavin Shaham. "Cheesecake-eating rats and the question of food addiction." *Nature Neuroscience* 13 (2010): 529–31.

"Evidence of Food Addiction." *Consumer Reports on Health* (July 2011): 2.

"Facing America's Obesity Crisis." *The Diane Rehm Show.* National Public Radio, May 10, 2012.

Fairburn, Christopher, and G. Terrence Wilson. *Binge Eating Disorder: Nature, Assessment and Treatment.* New York: Guilford Press, 1996.

"'Feel-good' food might be addictive." *Consumer Reports on Health* 10. Last modified November 2012. www.wellbeingjournal.com/vol-22-no-3-mayjune-2013/.

Flint, Alan, et al. "Food addiction scale measurement in 2 cohorts of middle-aged and older women." *American Journal of Clinical Nutrition*, 99, no. 3 (March 2014): 578–86.

"Forget Diet Pills, Try Oatmeal." *Good Morning America.* ABC News. December 2005.

Garner, David, et al. "A comparison of cognitive-behavioral and supportive-expressive therapy for bulimia nervosa." *American Journal of Psychiatry* 150, no. 1 (1993): 37–46.

Gearhardt, Ashley N., William R. Corbin, and Kelly D. Brownell. "Preliminary Validation of the Yale Food Addiction Scale." *Appetite* 52 (2008): 430–36.

Gearhardt, Ashley, Corbin, N., and Brownell, W.R. "Development of the Yale Food Addiction Scale Version 2.0." *Psychology of Addictive Behaviors* 30 no.1 (Feb 2016): 113-121.

Geier-Horan, A. "ASAM Releases New Definition of Addiction: Addiction Is a Chronic Brain Disease, Not Just Bad Behaviors or Bad Choices." Press release. American Society of Addiction Medicine. August 15, 2011.

Gerstein, D.R. "Treating Drug Problems." *New England Journal of Medicine* 323, no. 12 (September 20, 1990): 844–48.

Gilbert, P., et al. "Prevention and Treatment of Pediatric Obesity: An Endocrine Society Clinical Practice Guideline Based on Expert Opinion." *The Journal of Clinical Endocrinology and Metabolism*, 93, no. 12 (December 2008): 4576-4599.

Glasser, William. *Positive Addiction.* New York: Harper & Row, 1985.

Grant, J.E., et al. "Introduction to Behavioral Addictions." *American Journal of Drug and Alcohol Abuse* 36, no. 5 (2010): 233–41.

Gross, Michael. "Alcoholics Anonymous: Still sober after 75 years." *American Journal of Public Health* 100, no. 12 (2010): 2361–63.

Gudzune K.A., et al. "Efficacy of Commercial Weight-Loss Programs: An Updated Systematic Review." *Annals of Internal Medicine* 162, no.7 (April 7 2015): 501-12. doi: 10.7326/M14-2238.

Gupta, Sumati. "Is Bulimia Like a Drug Addiction?" Psychology Today. Last modified June 22, 2012. www.psychologytoday.com/blog/emotional-eating/201206/is-bulimia-drug-addiction.

Hari, Jonathan. "Everything You Think You Know about Addiction is Wrong." Filmed June 2015: at TedGlobalLondon, London, England. Video, 14:43. https://www.ted.com/talks/johann_hari_everything_you_think_you_know_about_addiction_is_wrong.

Harman, Pat. "Many Doctors Believe Food Can Be Addictive." Childhood Obesity News, Jan 27 2011. http://childhoodobesitynews.com/2011/01/27/many-doctors-believe- food-can-be-addictive.

Hartocollis, Anemona. "Young, Obese and In Surgery." *New York Times*, January 8, 2012.

Hay, P.J., J. Bacaltchuk. and S. Stefano. "Psychotherapy for bulimia nervosa and binging." *Cochrane Database of Systematic Reviews* 3 (2004): 1–73.

Hill, J., and R. Wing. "The National Weight Control Registry." *Permanente Journal* 7, no. 3 (Summer 2003): 34–37.

Hillock, C. "Outcome Research on ACORN Events." Paper presented to the Promising Practices Conference of the International Society of Food Addiction Professionals, Houston, Texas, January 2009.

Hollis, Judi. *Fat Is a Family Affair*. Center City, MN: Hazelden Foundation, 1985.

Hudson, J.I., et al. "The Prevalence and Correlates of Eating Disorders in the National Comorbidity Survey Replication." *Biological Psychiatry* 61, no. 3 (2007): 348–58.

Hyman, Steven E. "Addiction: A Disease of Learning and Memory." *American Journal of Psychiatry* 162, no. 8 (2005): 1414–22.

Ifland, Joan. *Sugars and Flours: How They Make Us Crazy, Sick and Fat and What to Do About It*. Bloomington, IN: AuthorHouse, 2003.

Ifland, Joan, et al. "Refined food addiction: A classic substance use disorder." *Medical Hypotheses* 72 (2009): 518–26.

Janssen, Imke, et al. "Testosterone and Visceral Fat in Midlife Women: The Study of Women's Health Across the Nation (SWAN) Fat Patterning Study." *Obesity* 18, no. 3 (March 2010): 604–10.

Jellinek, E.M. "Addiction and Recovery: The Jellinek Curve." www.in.gov/judiciary/ijlap/jellinek.pdf.

———. *The Disease Concept of Alcoholism*. New Haven, CT: Hillhouse, 1960.

Jenkins, A. "Consumed by an addiction." *Nursing Standard* 20, no. 29 (March 29, 2006): 32–33.

Johnson, Melinda. "The Diet Mentality Paradox: Why Dieting Can Make You Fat." U.S. News & World Report. Last modified August 17, 2012. http://health.usnews.com/health-news/blogs/eat-run/2012/08/17/the-diet-mentality-paradox-why-dieting-can-make-you-fat.

Johnson, P.M., and P.J. Kenny "Dopamine D2 receptors in addiction-like reward dysfunction and compulsive eating in obese rats." *Nature Neuroscience* 13, no. 5 (2010): 635–41.

Kasl, Charlotte. *Many Roads, One Journey: Moving Beyond the 12 Steps*. New York: HarperCollins, 1992.

Katherine, Anne. *Anatomy of a Food Addiction: The Brain Chemistry of Overeating*. Carlsbad, DE: Gurze Books, 1996.

Kessler, David. *The End of Overeating: Taking Control of the Insatiable American Appetite*. New York: Rodale, 2009.

———. *Your Food Is Fooling You: How Your Brain Is Hijacked by Sugar, Fat, and Salt*. New York: Roaring Brook Press, 2013.

"Kids' Sugar Cravings Might Be Biological." *Morning Edition*. National Public Radio, September 26, 2011.

King, Wendy C., et al. "Prevalence of Alcohol Use Disorders Before and After Bariatric Surgery." *Journal of the American Medical Association* 307, no. 23 (June 2012): 2516–25.

Klein, D.A., et al. "Artificial sweetener use among individuals with eating disorders." *International Journal of Eating Disorders* 39, no. 4 (2006): 341–45.

Klok, M.D., S. Jakobsdottir, and M.L. Drent. "The role of leptin and ghrelin in the regulation of food intake and body weight in humans: a review." *Obesity Reviews* 8, no. 1 (2007): 21–34.

Kluger, J., and E. Dias. "Does God Want You to Be Thin?" *Time* (June 11, 2012): 41–49.

Kolata, Gina. "Study Shows Why It's Hard to Keep Weight Off." *New York Times*, October 27, 2011.

Kubler-Ross, Elizabeth. *On Death and Dying.* New York: Scribner, 1969.

Kurtz, Ernest. *Not-God: A History of Alcoholics Anonymous.* Center City, MN: Hazelden Educational Materials, 1979.

Lee, C. "The Sex Addiction Epidemic." *Newsweek* (December 5, 2011).

Leibowitz, Sarah F. "Mechanisms of Food Cravings." Paper presented to the Obesity and Food Addiction Summit, IslandWood, Bainbridge Island, WA, April 25, 2009.

———. "Overconsumption of dietary fat and alcohol: Mechanisms involving lipids and hypothalamic peptides." *Physiology & Behavior* 91, no. 5 (2007): 513–21.

Lenoir, Magalie, et al. "Intense Sweetness Surpasses Cocaine Reward." *PLoS ONE* 2, no. 8 (2007): 698.

Levitan, R.D., and C.A. Davis. "Emotions and Eating Behaviour: Implications for the Current Obesity Epidemic." *University of Toronto Quarterly* 79, no. 2 (2010): 783–99.

Liebman, Bonnie. "Food & Addiction: Can Some Foods Hijack the Brain?" *Nutrition Action Healthletter* (May 2012): 3–7.

———. "Fooled by Food." *Nutrition Action Healthletter* (April 2013): 3–7.

Linden, David. *The Compass of Pleasure: How Our Brains Make Fatty Foods, Orgasm, Exercise, Marijuana, Generosity, Vodka, Learning and Gambling Feel So Good.* New York: Penguin Books, 2014.

Lisle, D. J. *The Pleasure Trap: Mastering the Hidden Forces that Undermine Health and Happiness.* Kobo, Book Publishing Company, 2003.

Loewen, Stanley. "Addictive Personality Disorder." HealthGuidance.org. www.health-guidance.org/entry/15805/1/Addictive-Personality-Disorder.html.

"Lose weight your way: 9,000 readers rate 13 diet plans and tools." *Consumer Reports* (February 2013): 26–28.

Lustig, Robert H. *Fat Chance: Beating the Odds Against Sugar, Processed Food, Obesity, and Disease.* New York: Penguin Plume, 2012.

———. *The Hacking of the American Mind: The Science Behind the Corporate Takeover of Our Bodies and our Brains.* New York: Penguin Random House, 2017.

Maleskey, G. "Addicted to Sugar?" *SpryLiving* 7 (June 2012).

Maté, Gabor. *In the Realm of the Hungry Ghosts: Close Encounters with Addiction.* Berkeley, CA: North Atlantic Books, 2010.

McAleavey, K. I. "Ten Years of Treating Eating Disorders: What Have We Learned? A Personal Perspective on the Application of the 12 step and Wellness Programs." *Advances in Mind-Body Medicine.* 23, no. 2 (Summer 2008): 18–26.

McCoy (Rigby), C. "A Onetime Olympic Gymnast Overcomes the Bulimia That Threatened Her Life." *People* (August 13, 1984): 68–72.

Megan, B. "Nonnutritive Sweeteners and Cardio-metabolic Health: A Systemic Review and Meta-analysis of Randomized Controlled Trials and Prospective Cohort Studies." *CMAJ,* 189, no. 28 (July 2017): E929-E939. https://doi.org/10.1503/cmaj.161390.

Meule, Adrian. "How Prevalent is 'Food Addiction?" *Frontiers in Psychiatry* 2, no. 61 (2011).

"Models at Risk for Eating Disorders." Eating Disorders Review. Last modified October, 2008. www.eatingdisordersreview.com/nl/nl_edr_19_5_6.html.

Morton, Andrew. *Diana: Her True Story in Her Own Words.* New York: Simon & Schuster, 1997.

Moss, Michael. *Salt, Sugar, Fat: How the Food Giants Hooked Us.* New York: Random House, 2013.

Munhall, Patricia. "Women's Anger and its meanings: A phenomeno-logical perspective." *Health Care for Women International* 14, no. 6 (2009): 481–91.

National Center on Addiction and Substance Abuse. *Understanding and Addressing Food Addiction: A Science Based Approach to Policy, Practice and Research,* Feb 2016.

National Institute on Drug Abuse. "Sight, Smell of Favorite Foods Are Related to Drug Craving." *NewsScan,* January 10, 2005.

NEDA (National Eating Disorder Association): Feeding Hope. Statistics and research on Eating Disorders. https://www.nationaleatingdisorders. org/statistics-research-eating-disorders.

Noble, E.P., et al. "D2 dopamine receptor gene and obesity." *International Journal of Eating Disorders* 15 (1994): 205–17.

Oaklander, Mandy. "10 Sneaky Names for Sugar." Prevention. Last modified October, 2012. www.prevention.com/food/healthy-eating-tips/ agave-glucose-and-other-names-sugar.

"The Obesity Epidemic." National Center for Chronic Disease Prevention and Health Promotion, Division of Nutrition, Physical Activity and Obesity. Last modified July 22, 2011. www.cdc.gov/cdtv.

Oglethorpe, Alice, and Noelle Howey. "The Facts About Emotional Eating." Real Simple. Last modified August 24, 2013. www.realsimple. com/health/mind-mood/emotional-health/emotional-eating-001000 00085639/index.html.

Okasaka, Y., et al. "Correlation between addictive behaviors and mental health in university students." *Psychiatry and Clinical Neurosciences* 62 (2008): 84–92.

Overeaters Anonymous. *Overeaters Anonymous.* Torrance, CA: Overeaters Anonymous, 2001.

———. *The Twelve Steps and Twelve Traditions of Overeaters Anonymous.* Torrance, CA: Overeaters Anonymous, 2010.

Papadopoulos, et al. "Excess mortality causes of death and prognostic factors in anorexia nervosa." *British Journal of Psychiatry* 194 (2009): 10–17.

Park, Alice. "Gym vs. Genes." Time. Last modified November 02, 2011. http://health-land.time.com/2011/11/02/gym-vs-genes-how- exercise-trumps-obesity-genes.

Peeke, Pamela, and Mariska van Aalst. *The Hunger Fix: The Three-Stage Detox and Recovery Plan for Overeating and Food Addiction.* Emmaus, PA: Rodale, 2012.

Peele, Stanton. "War Over Addiction: Evaluating The DSM-V." Huffington Post. Last modified February 11, 2010. www.huffingtonpost.com/ stanton-peele/war-over-addic- tion-evalua_b_456321.html.

Pepino, M. Yanina, et al. "Sucralose Affects Glycemic and Hormonal

Responses to an Oral Glucose Load." *Diabetes Care* 36, no. 9 (September 2013): 2530–35.

Phinney, Stephen, and Jeff Volek. "The Art and Science of Low Carbohydrate Living." Self-published, 2012.

Prager, Michael. *Fat Boy, Thin Man.* Fisherblue Press, 2010.

Price, M. "Genes matter in addiction." *Monitor* 39, no. 6 (2008): 14.

Puthenedam, Manjula. "PET imaging shows fewer dopamine receptors in drug addicts." *Health Imaging.* Last modified April 28, 2010. www.healthimaging.com/topics/molecular-imaging/study-pet-imaging-shows-fewer-dopamine-receptors-drug-addicts.

Rada, Pedro, et al. "A High-Fat meal, or Intraperitoneal Administration of a Fat Emulsion, Increases Extracellular Dopamine in the Nucleus Accumbens." *Brain Sciences* 2, no. 2 (June 11, 2012): 242–53.

Recitas, Lyn-Genet. *The Plan: Eliminate the Surprising "Healthy" Foods That Are Making You Fat — and Lose Weight Fast.* London: Orion Publishing, 2013.

Roth, Geneen. *Feeding the Hungry Heart: The Experience of Compulsive Eating.* New York: Penguin, 1993.

———. *Women, Food and God: An Unexpected Path to Almost Everything.* New York: Scribner, 2011.

Sack, David. "Where Science Meets the Steps: Why the Hostility Toward the 12 Steps?" Psychology Today. Last modified November 20, 2012. www.psychologytoday.com/ blog/where-science-meets-the-steps/201211/why-the-hostility-toward-the-12-steps.

Sacks, Fiona M. et al., "Comparison of Weight Loss Diets with Different Compositions of Fat, Protein, and Carbohydrates." *New England Journal of Medicine* 360, no. 9 (2009): 859–73.

Schatzker, Mark. *The Dorito Effect: The Surprising New Truth about Food and Flavor.* Simon and Schuster, 2015.

Schele, E., ed. "Does Food Addiction Exist?" NeuroFast.eu. Last modified December 12, 2012. www.neurofast.eu/science-for-all/does-food-addiction-exist/.

Science Daily – Science News. "Compulsive Eating shares addictive biochemical mechanism with Cocaine, Heroin Abuse, Study Shows." Scripps Research Institute, March 29, 2010.

Shalev, U., J. Yap, and Y. Shaham. "Leptin Attenuates Acute Food Deprivation-Induced Relapse to Heroin Seeking." *Journal of Neuroscience* 21, no. 4 (2001): RC129.

Shell, Ellen Ruppel. *The Hungry Gene: The Science of Fat and the Future of Thin.* New York: Atlantic Monthly Press Books, 2002.

Sheppard, Kay. *Food Addiction: The Body Knows.* Deerfield Beach, FL: Health Communications, 1993.

Shetty, P. "Nora Volkow — challenging the myths about drug addiction." *Lancet* 378, no. 9790 (2011): 477.

Silverglade, Bruce, and Ilene Ringel Heller. "Food Labeling Chaos, The Case for Reform." Center for Science in the Public Interest. Last modified 2010. www.cspinet.org/new/pdf/food_labeling_chaos_report.pdf.

"Similarities between obesity and addiction under study at NIDA." *Alcoholism & Drug Abuse Weekly* (June 4, 2007): 4–5.

Smith K.E., et al. "Problematic Alcohol Use and Associated Characteristics Following Bariatric Surgery." *Obesity Surgery.* 2017.

Spring, Bonnie, et al. "Abuse potential of carbohydrates for overweight carbohydrate cravers." *Psychopharmacology* 197 (2008): 637–47.

Stewart, T.M., D.A. Williamson, and M.A. White. "Rigid vs. flexible dieting: association with eating disorder symptoms in non-obese women." *Appetite* 38, no. 1 (2002): 39–44.

Sumithran, Priya, et al. "Long-Term Persistence of Hormonal Adaptations to Weight Loss." *New England Journal of Medicine* 365 (2011): 1597–1604.

Szalavitz, Maia. "Can Eating Junk Food Really Be an Addiction?" Time. Last modified April 03, 2010. http://content.time.com/time/health/article/0,8599,1977604,00.html.

Tarman, Vera. *Dangerous Liaisons: Comfort and Food — Understand Food Addiction.* Lecture. Toronto: Addictions Unplugged, 2013. DVD.

———. *Food Addiction: Addictions Unplugged, Why We Get Wired, and How to Unplug.* Lecture, Toronto: Addictions Unplugged, 2013. DVD.

———. "Food Addiction/Sugar Addiction Expert Forum." Medhelp. Last modified 2012. www.medhelp.org.

Taubes, Gary. *The Case Against Sugar,* New York: Alfred A. Knofp, 2016.

———. "The New Obesity Campaigns Have It All Wrong." *Newsweek* (May 14, 2012): 32–36.

Thanos, P.K., et al. "Food restriction markedly increases dopamine D2 receptor (D2R) in a rat model of obesity as assessed with in-vivo muPET imaging." *Synapse* 62, no. 1 (January 2008): 50–61.

Toedtman, Jim. "Tax Attack: Higher taxes have discouraged public consumption of whiskey and tobacco. Now it's sugar's turn." *AARP Bulletin* (June 2012): 3.

Treuhaft, S., and A. Karpyn. *The Grocery Gap: Who Has Access to Healthy Food and Why It Matters.* Study. PolicyLink and The Food Trust, March 15, 2010.

Twenty-Four Hours a Day. Center City, MN: Hazelden Educational Materials, Town Hall, Los Angeles, CA, April 27, 2006.

Trimpey, Jack. *The Small Book: A Revolutionary Alternative for Overcoming Alcohol and Drug Dependence (Rational Recovery Systems).* Dell, 1055.

U.S. News & World Report. "Information on Bariatric Surgery." Last modified January 2010. https://health.usnews.com/health-conditions/ heart-health/information-on-bariatric-surgery/overview.

Vassallo, Tony. *Weight Loss Never Tasted so Good Cookbook, 2nd ed.* Toronto, Create Space, 2017.

Voigt, Deborah. *Call me Debby: True Confessions of a Down to Earth Diva.* Harper, 2015.

———. "New Vaccines Are Being Developed Against Addiction and Relapse." *NIDA Notes* 22 (2008): 2.

Volkow, Nora D., and T-K Li. "Drug addiction: the neurobiology of behaviour gone awry." *Neuroscience* 5 (2004): 963–70.

Volkow, Nora D., and Roy A. Wise. "How can drug addiction help us understand obesity?" *Nature Neuroscience* 8, no. 5 (2005): 555–60.

Volkow, Nora D., et al. "The Addictive Dimensionality of Obesity." *Biological Psychiatry* 73 (2013): 811–18.

———. "Imaging the neurochemistry of nicotine actions: studies with positron emission tomography." *Nicotine & Tobacco Research* 1 (1999): S127–S132.

———. "Low Level of Brain Dopamine D2 Receptors in Methamphetamine Abusers: Association with Metabolism in the Orbitofrontal Cortex." *American Psychiatric Association Focus* 1 (2003): 150–57.

———. "Pro v Con Reviews: Is Food Addictive? Obesity and Addiction: Neurobiological Overlaps." Obes Review 2013, Jan: 14 (1) 2–18.

Walls, Helen L., et al. "Public health campaigns and obesity — a critique." *BMC Public Health* 11 (2011): 136.

Wang, Gene-Jack, et al. "Brain dopamine and obesity." *Lancet* 357 (2001): 354–57.

———. "Similarity Between Obesity and Drug Addiction as Assessed by Neurofunctional Imaging: A Concept Review." *Journal of Addictive Diseases* 23 (2004): 39–53.

Wansink, Brian. *Mindless Eating — Why We Eat More Than We Think.* New York: Bantam Books, 2010.

"Weight Loss Surgery Increases Risk of Alcohol Addiction." *Good Morning America.* ABC News. Last modified June 2012. www.abcnews.go.com/Health/Wellness.

"Weighty Issues: World's heaviest countries." *Time* (July 9, 2012).

Werdell, Philip. *Bariatric Surgery & Food Addiction: Preoperative Considerations.* Sarasota, FL: EverGreen Publications, 2009.

Weltens, N., et al. *Food Addiction Recovery, A New Model of Professional Support: The ACORN Primary Intensive.* Sarasota, FL: EverGreen Publications, 2007.

———. "Where is the Comfort in Comfort Foods? Mechanisms linking Fat Singling, Reward and Emotion. Review Article." *Neurogastroenterology and Motility* (2014), 26: 303–15.

Wideman, C.H., G.R. Nadzam, and H.M. Murphy. "Implications of an Animal Model of Sugar Addiction, Withdrawal, and Relapse for Human Health." *Nutritional Neuroscience* 8, nos. 5–6 (2005): 269–76.

Wilson, T.G. "Current Status of Behavioral Treatment of Obesity." In *Behavioral Analysis and Treatment of Substance Abuse*, edited by N.A. Krasnegor, 202–23. Rockville, MD: National Institute on Drug Abuse, Division of Research, 1979.

Woods, S.C. "Gastrointestinal Satiety Signals: An overview of gastrointestinal signals that influence food intake." *Journal of Physiology* 286, no. 1 (2004): G7–G13.

Zuger, Abigail. "A General in the Drug War." *New York Times*, June 14, 2011.

INDEX

CPSIA information can be obtained
at www.ICGtesting.com
Printed in the USA
JSHW031518290921
19144JS00003B/53